In memory of Daniel X. Freedman, mentor, colleague, and scientific father.

To Cindy, my wife, best friend, and tireless supporter.

To Jennifer and Victoria, my daughters, for their patience and understanding of the demands of authorship.

Antipsychotics and Mood Stabilizers

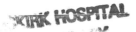
The best-selling *Stahl's Essential Psychopharmacology* – fully revised and updated throughout – continues its tradition of being the preeminent source of information in its field. More than one-third longer than the previous edition, this third edition of *Antipsychotics and Mood Stabilizers* draws from the revised chapters in *Stahl's Essential Psychopharmacology* to form a resource that is essential reading for all clinicians treating psychosis as well as for all students who need to know the mechanisms of drug actions. Straightforward and eminently readable, this edition can be read cover to cover by experts and novices alike.

Stephen M. Stahl is Adjunct Professor of Psychiatry at the University of California at San Diego. He has conducted numerous research projects awarded by the National Institute of Mental Health, the Veterans Administration, and the pharmaceutical industry. Author of more than 350 articles and chapters, Dr. Stahl is an internationally recognized clinician, researcher, and teacher in psychiatry with subspecialty expertise in psychopharmacology.

Antipsychotics and Mood Stabilizers

Stahl's Essential Psychopharmacology

Third Edition

Stephen M. Stahl

University of California at San Diego

With Illustrations by
Nancy Muntner

Editorial Assistant
Meghan M. Grady

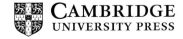

CAMBRIDGE
UNIVERSITY PRESS

CAMBRIDGE UNIVERSITY PRESS
Cambridge, New York, Melbourne, Madrid, Cape Town, Singapore, São Paulo, Delhi

Cambridge University Press
32 Avenue of the Americas, New York, NY 10013-2473, USA

www.cambridge.org
Information on this title: www.cambridge.org/9780521714136

First published 2008

Printed in the United States of America

A catalog record for this publication is available from the British Library.

Library of Congress Cataloging in Publication Data

Stahl, S. M.
    Antipsychotics and mood stabilizers : Stahl's essential
psychopharmacology, 3rd edition / Stephen M. Stahl ; with illustrations by
Nancy Muntner.
      p. ; cm.
    Includes index.
    ISBN 978-0-521-88664-2 (hardback) – ISBN 978-0-521-71413-6 (pbk.)
    1. Antipsychotic drugs–Handbooks, manuals, etc.   2. Affective
disorders–Chemotherapy–Handbooks, manuals, etc.   3. Psychoses–Chemotherapy–Handbooks,
manuals, etc.   I. Stahl, S. M. Stahl's essential psychopharmacology.   II. Title.
    [DNLM: 1. Antipsychotic Agents–pharmacology.   2. Mood Disorders–drug
therapy.   3. Schizophrenia–drug therapy. QV 77.9 S781a 2008]
    RM333.5.S7338 2008
    615′.7882–dc22
                                                                          2008004352

ISBN 978-0-521-88664-2   hardback
ISBN 978-0-521-71413-6   paperback

Contents

Preface to the Third Edition

This booklet is a set of the two chapters from the third edition of *Stahl's Essential Psychopharmacology* that deal exclusively with psychosis and schizophrenia and their treatment with antipsychotic drugs. The knowledge base of psychopharmacology for psychosis and schizophrenia has expanded considerably since publication of the second edition of this book, and the third edition attempts to reflect these changes.

In most developed countries, antipsychotics have become the most expensive therapeutic market, not only for psychiatry, but for medical therapeutics in general. Since prescribers are rapidly expanding their utilization of the newer antipsychotics for the treatment of disorders other than psychosis, such as for the treatment of bipolar disorder and various treatment-resistant disorders of anxiety and mood, it is particularly important to understand how the drugs categorized here as "antipsychotics" work. This therapeutic area of psychopharmacology occupies one of the largest sections of the full textbook and is perhaps the section that has undergone the most change since publication of the second edition. Given the importance of this area of psychopharmacology, many readers may be interested in this area alone; therefore, we offer the two chapters on psychosis and on antipsychotics as a stand-alone spinoff of the third edition of *Stahl's Essential Psychopharmacology*.

Psychopharmacology has not only experienced incredible growth since publication of the second edition of this textbook; it has also experienced a major paradigm shift from a limited focus on neurotransmitters and receptors to an emphasis as well on brain circuits, neuroimaging, genetics, and signal transduction cascades. The third edition of *Stahl's Essential Psychopharmacology* attempts to reflect this transformation in the field, and elements of this paradigm shift are incorporated into each of these chapters in this booklet. Many new antipsychotics have been introduced in recent years, and many more are now in clinical testing, and these are covered in this new edition. These two chapters on psychosis and antipsychotics have been extensively reorganized, rewritten, and illustrated with roughly twice the number of figures in every chapter. However, what has not changed is the didactic style of the first and second editions, which continues in this third edition.

The text is purposely written at a conceptual level rather than a pragmatic level and includes ideas that are simplifications and rules, while sacrificing precision and discussion of exceptions to rules. Thus, this is not a text intended for the sophisticated subspecialist in psychopharmacology. Also, it is not extensively referenced to original papers, but rather to textbooks and reviews and a few selected original papers, with only a limited reading list for each chapter. For those of you interested in specific prescribing information about the most common one hundred or so psychotropic drugs, this information is available in the companion textbook, *Essential Psychopharmacology Prescriber's Guide*. A spinoff of this book just on antipsychotics (and mood stabilizers) is also available, called *Essential Psychopharmacology Prescriber's Guide of Antipsychotics and Mood Stabilizers*.

Now, you also have the option of going to Essential Psychopharmacology Online at www.essentialpsych.org. We are proud to announce the launch of this new website, which is due to premiere in the fall of 2008. Access to this website will allow you to search within the entire Essential Psychopharmacology series that includes not only the third edition of *Stahl's Essential Psychopharmacology*, but also *Essential Psychopharmacology Prescriber's Guide*. This site will be updated regularly and should therefore provide an up-to-date source for what you need to know about the essentials of psychopharmacology between publication of subsequent editions of these books.

Much of the new content in this text is based on updated lectures, courses, slides, and articles by the author. Many of the new illustrations are now available as animations on the Neuroscience Education Institute's website, as are the lectures, slides and articles, continuing medical education (CME) credits, tests, certifications, and much more. I invite you to explore this interactive reference by visiting the Neuroscience Education Institute's website at www.neiglobal.com. If you are interested in comprehensive materials, you can choose to have access to both websites.

In general, this text attempts to present the fundamentals of psychopharmacology in simplified and readily readable form. Thus, this material should prepare the reader to consult more sophisticated textbooks as well as the professional literature. The organization of the information here also applies principles of programmed learning for the reader, namely repetition and interaction, which has been shown to enhance retention.

Therefore, it is suggested that novices first approach this text by going through it from beginning to end, reviewing only the color graphics and the legends for these graphics. Virtually everything covered in the text is also covered in the graphics and icons. Once having gone through all the color graphics in these chapters, it is recommended that the reader then go back to the beginning of the book and read the entire text, reviewing the graphics at the same time. After the text has been read, the entire book can be rapidly reviewed again merely by referring to the various color graphics in the book. Finally, as a member of the Neuroscience Education Institute, you can utilize the content available online at www.neiglobal.com to obtain continuing medical education credits for this activity or as a helpful interactive reference. Many of the graphics are animated and available on this site. Also, you can search topics in the field covered in the Essential Psychopharmacology book series on Essential Psychopharmacology Online.

This mechanism of using the materials will create a certain amount of programmed learning by incorporating the elements of repetition, as well as interaction with visual learning through graphics. Hopefully, the visual concepts learned via graphics will reinforce abstract concepts learned from the written text, especially for those of you who are primarily "visual learners" (i.e., those who retain information better from visualizing concepts than from reading about them).

For those of you who are already familiar with psychopharmacology, this book should provide easy reading from beginning to end. Going back and forth between the text and the graphics should provide interaction. Following review of the complete text, it should be simple to review the entire book by going through the graphics once again. In addition, the Neuroscience Education Institute's website further expands the Essential Psychopharmacology learning experience and Essential Psychopharmacology Online allows quick searches of topics in this field.

For those of you interested in the specific updates made in the third edition, the psychosis chapter has much expanded coverage of the neurotransmitter glutamate and of the interactions among glutamate, serotonin, and dopamine. The NMDA (N-methyl-d-aspartate) receptor hypofunction hypothesis of schizophrenia is extensively discussed, as are the various genetic advances occurring in schizophrenia research. Included are sections on matching the symptoms of psychosis and schizophrenia to various hypothetically malfunctioning brain circuits. Several new antipsychotics are also included in this third edition, as well numerous new agents of novel mechanism on the horizon for the treatment of psychosis and schizophrenia. There is extensive coverage of cardiometabolic risks and sedation related to antipsychotics, particularly certain of the newer atypical antipsychotics.

This is an incredibly exciting time for the fields of neuroscience and mental health, creating fascinating opportunities for clinicians to utilize current therapeutics and to anticipate future medications that are likely to transform the field of psychopharmacology. Best wishes for your first step on your journey into this fascinating field of psychopharmacology.

Stephen M. Stahl, M.D, Ph.D.

CME Information

Release/Expiration Dates

Original release date: March 2008
CME credit expiration date: original expiration February 2011 (if this date has passed, please contact NEI for updated information)

Target Audience

This activity was designed for health care professionals, including psychiatrists, neurologists, primary care physicians, pharmacists, psychologists, nurses, and others, who treat patients with psychiatric conditions.

Statement of Need

The content of this educational activity was determined by rigorous assessment, including activity feedback, expert faculty assessment, literature review, and new medical knowledge, which revealed the following unmet needs:

- Psychiatric illnesses such as schizophrenia have a neurobiological basis and are primarily treated by pharmacological agents; understanding each of these, as well as the relationship between them, is essential in order to select appropriate treatment for a patient

- The field of psychopharmacology has experienced incredible growth; it has also experienced a major paradigm shift from a limited focus on neurotransmitters and receptors to an emphasis as well on brain circuits, neuroimaging, genetics, and signal transduction cascades

Learning Objectives

Upon completion of this activity, you should be able to:

- Apply neurobiologic and mechanistic evidence when selecting treatment strategies in order to match treatment to the individual needs of the patient

- Utilize new scientific data to modify existing treatment strategies in order to improve patient outcomes in schizophrenia

Accreditation and Credit Designation Statements

The Neuroscience Education Institute is accredited by the Accreditation Council for Continuing Medical Education to provide continuing medical education for physicians.

The Neuroscience Education Institute designates this educational activity for a maximum of 16.0 *AMA PRA Category 1 Credits*™. Physicians should only claim credit commensurate with the extent of their participation in the activity.

Activity Instructions

This CME activity is in the form of a printed book and incorporates instructional design to enhance your retention of the information and pharmacological concepts that are being presented. You are advised to go through the figures in this activity from beginning to end, followed by the text, and then complete the posttests and evaluations. The estimated time for completion of this activity is 16 hours.

Instructions for CME Credit

To receive a certificate of CME credit or participation, please complete the posttest (you must score at least 70% to receive credit) and evaluation available online only at http://www .neiglobal.com/ep3. If a score of 70% or more is attained, you can immediately print your certificate. There is a fee for the posttest (certificate included) for non-NEI members.

NEI Disclosure Policy

It is the policy of the Neuroscience Education Institute to ensure balance, independence, objectivity, and scientific rigor in its educational activities. The Neuroscience Education Institute takes responsibility for the content, quality, and scientific integrity of this CME activity.

All faculty participating in any NEI-sponsored educational activity and all individuals in a position to influence or control content development are required by NEI to disclose to the activity audience any financial relationships or apparent conflicts of interest that may have a direct bearing on the subject matter of the activity. Although potential conflicts of interest are identified and resolved prior to the activity, it remains for the audience to determine whether outside interests reflect a possible bias in either the exposition or the conclusions presented.

Neither the Neuroscience Education Institute nor Stephen M. Stahl, MD, PhD has received any funds or grants in support of this educational activity.

Individual Disclosure Statements

Authors/Developers
Stephen M. Stahl, MD, PhD
Adjunct Professor, Department of Psychiatry
University of California, San Diego School of Medicine, San Diego, CA

Dr. Stahl has been a consultant, board member, or on the speakers bureau for the following pharmaceutical companies within the last three years: Acadia, Alkermes, Amylin, Asahi Kasei, Astra Zeneca, Avera, Azur, Biovail, Boehringer Ingelheim, BristolMyers Squibb, Cephalon, CSC Pharmaceuticals, Cyberonics, Cypress Bioscience, Dainippon, Eli Lilly, Forest, GlaxoSmithKline, Janssen, Jazz Pharmaceuticals, Labopharm, Lundbeck, Neurocrine Biosciences, NeuroMolecular, Neuronetics, Novartis, Organon, Pamlab, Pfizer, Pierre Fabre, sanofi-aventis, Schering-Plough, Sepracor, Shire, SK Corporation, Solvay, Somaxon, Takeda, Tethys, Tetragenix, Vanda Pharmaceuticals, and Wyeth.

Meghan Grady
Director, Content Development
Neuroscience Education Institute, Carlsbad, CA

No other financial relationships to disclose.

Editorial and Design Staff
Nancy Muntner
Director, Medical Illustrations
Neuroscience Education Institute, Carlsbad, CA

No other financial relationships to disclose.

Disclosed financial relationships have been reviewed by the Neuroscience Education Institute CME Advisory Board to resolve any potential conflicts of interest. All faculty and planning committee members have attested that their financial relationships do not affect their ability to present well-balanced, evidence-based content for this activity.

Disclosure of Off-Label Use

This educational activity may include discussion of unlabeled and/or investigational uses of agents that are not approved by the FDA. Please consult the product prescribing information for full disclosure of labeled uses.

Disclaimer

Participants have an implied responsibility to use the newly acquired information from this activity to enhance patient outcomes and their own professional development. The information presented in this educational activity is not meant to serve as a guideline for patient management. Any procedures, medications, or other courses of diagnosis or treatment discussed or suggested in this educational activity should not be used by clinicians without evaluation of their patients' conditions and possible contraindications or dangers in use, review of any applicable manufacturer's product information, and comparison with recommendations of other authorities. Primary references and full prescribing information should be consulted.

Sponsorship Information

Sponsored by Neuroscience Education Institute

Support

This activity is supported solely by the sponsor, Neuroscience Education Institute.

Psychosis and Schizophrenia

Psychosis is a difficult term to define and is frequently misused, not only in the newspapers, in movies, and on television but unfortunately among mental health professionals as well. Stigma and fear surround the concept of psychosis, and the average citizen worries about long-standing myths of "mental illness," including "psychotic killers," "psychotic rage," and the equivalence of "psychosis" with the pejorative term "crazy."

There is perhaps no area of psychiatry where misconceptions are greater than in that of psychotic illnesses. The reader is well served to develop an expertise on the facts about the diagnosis and treatment of psychotic illnesses in order to dispel unwarranted beliefs and to help destigmatize this devastating group of illnesses. This chapter is not intended to list the diagnostic criteria for all the different mental disorders of which psychosis is either a defining or associated feature. The reader is referred to standard reference sources (DSM-IV and ICD-10) for that information. Although schizophrenia is emphasized here, we will approach psychosis as a syndrome associated with a variety of illnesses that are all targets for antipsychotic drug treatment.

Symptom dimensions in schizophrenia

Clinical description of psychosis

Psychosis is a syndrome – a mixture of symptoms – that can be associated with many different psychiatric disorders, but it is not a specific disorder itself in diagnostic schemes such as DSM-IV or ICD-10. At a minimum, psychosis means delusions and hallucinations. It generally also includes symptoms such as disorganized speech, disorganized behavior, and gross distortions of reality testing.

Therefore psychosis can be considered to be a set of symptoms in which a person's mental capacity, affective response, and capacity to recognize reality, communicate, and relate to others is impaired. Psychotic disorders have psychotic symptoms as their defining features; there are, however, other disorders in which psychotic symptoms may be present but are not necessary for the diagnosis.

Those **disorders that require the presence of psychosis** as a *defining* feature of the diagnosis include schizophrenia, substance-induced (i.e., drug-induced) psychotic disorder, schizophreniform disorder, schizoaffective disorder, delusional disorder, brief psychotic disorder, shared psychotic disorder, and psychotic disorder due to a general medical condition (Table 1-1). **Disorders that may or may not have psychotic symptoms** as an *associated* feature include mania and depression as well as several cognitive disorders such as Alzheimer's dementia (Table 1-2).

Psychosis itself can be paranoid, disorganized/excited, or depressive. Perceptual distortions and motor disturbances can be associated with any type of psychosis. **Perceptual distortions** include being distressed by hallucinatory voices; hearing voices that accuse, blame, or threaten punishment; seeing visions; reporting hallucinations of touch, taste, or odor; or reporting that familiar things and people seem changed. **Motor disturbances** are peculiar, rigid postures; overt signs of tension; inappropriate grins or giggles; peculiar

TABLE 1-1 Disorders in which psychosis is a defining feature

Schizophrenia
Substance-induced (i.e., drug-induced) psychotic disorders
Schizophreniform disorder
Schizoaffective disorder
Delusional disorder
Brief psychotic disorder
Shared psychotic disorder
Psychotic disorder due to a general medical condition

TABLE 1-2 Disorders in which psychosis is an associated feature

Mania
Depression
Cognitive disorders
Alzheimer's dementia

repetitive gestures; talking, muttering, or mumbling to oneself; or glancing around as if hearing voices.

In **paranoid psychosis**, the patient has paranoid projections, hostile belligerence, and grandiose expansiveness. **Paranoid projection** includes preoccupation with delusional beliefs; believing that people are talking about oneself; believing one is being persecuted or being conspired against; and believing that people or external forces control one's actions. **Hostile belligerence** is a verbal expression of feelings of hostility; expressing an attitude of disdain; manifesting a hostile, sullen attitude; manifesting irritability and grouchiness; tending to blame others for problems; expressing feelings of resentment; complaining and finding fault; as well as expressing suspicion of people. **Grandiose expansiveness** is exhibiting an attitude of superiority; hearing voices that praise and extol; and believing one has unusual powers, is a well known personality, or has a divine mission.

In a **disorganized/excited psychosis**, there is conceptual disorganization, disorientation, and excitement. **Conceptual disorganization** can be characterized by giving answers that are irrelevant or incoherent, drifting off the subject, using neologisms, or repeating certain words or phrases. **Disorientation** is not knowing where one is, the season of the year, the calendar year, or one's own age. **Excitement** is expressing feelings without restraint, manifesting speech that is hurried, exhibiting an elevated mood, showing an attitude of superiority, dramatizing oneself or one's symptoms, manifesting loud and boisterous speech, exhibiting overactivity or restlessness, and exhibiting excess of speech.

Depressive psychosis is characterized by retardation, apathy, and anxious self-punishment and blame. **Retardation and apathy** are manifesting slowed speech, indifference to one's future, fixed facial expression, slowed movements, deficiencies in recent memory, blocking in speech, apathy toward oneself or one's problems, slovenly appearance, low or whispered speech, and failure to answer questions. **Anxious self-punishment and blame** is the tendency to blame or condemn oneself; anxiety about specific matters; apprehensiveness regarding vague future events; an attitude of self-deprecation; manifesting a depressed mood; expressing feelings of guilt and remorse; preoccupation with suicidal thoughts, unwanted ideas, and specific fears; and feeling unworthy or sinful.

This discussion of clusters of psychotic symptoms does not constitute diagnostic criteria for any psychotic disorder. It is given merely as a description of several types of symptoms in psychosis to give the reader an overview of the nature of behavioral disturbances associated with the various psychotic illnesses.

Schizophrenia is more than a psychosis

Although schizophrenia is the commonest and best known psychotic illness, it is not synonymous with psychosis but is just one of many causes of psychosis. Schizophrenia affects 1 percent of the population, and in the United States there are over 300,000 acute schizophrenic episodes annually. Between 25 and 50 percent of schizophrenia patients

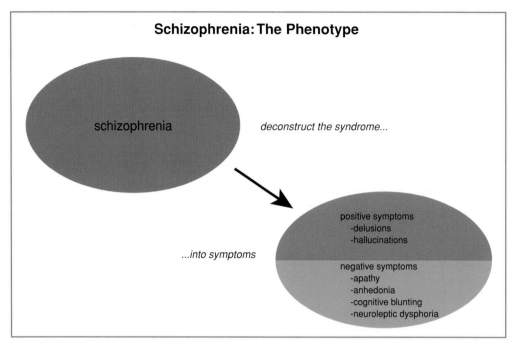

FIGURE 1-1 Positive and negative symptoms. The syndrome of schizophrenia consists of a mixture of symptoms that are commonly divided into two major categories, positive and negative. Positive symptoms, such as delusions and hallucinations, reflect the development of the symptoms of psychosis; they can be dramatic and may reflect loss of touch with reality. Negative symptoms reflect the loss of normal functions and feelings, such as losing interest in things and not being able to experience pleasure.

attempt suicide, and 10 percent eventually succeed, contributing to a mortality rate eight times greater than that of the general population. The life expectancy of a schizophrenic patient may be 20 to 30 years shorter than that of the general population, not only due to suicide but in particular due to premature cardiovascular disease. Accelerated mortality from premature cardiovascular disease in schizophrenic patients is caused not only by genetic factors and lifestyle choices – such as smoking, unhealthy diet, and lack of exercise leading to obesity and diabetes – but also, unfortunately, by treatment with some antipsychotic drugs, which themselves cause an increased incidence of obesity and diabetes and thus increased cardiac risk. In the United States, over 20 percent of all social security benefit days are used for the care of schizophrenic patients. The direct and indirect costs of schizophrenia in the United States alone are estimated to be in the tens of billions of dollars every year.

Schizophrenia by definition is a disturbance that must last for 6 months or longer, including at least 1 month of delusions, hallucinations, disorganized speech, grossly disorganized or catatonic behavior, or negative symptoms. Thus, symptoms of schizophrenia are often divided into positive and negative symptoms (Figure 1-1).

Positive symptoms are listed in Table 1-3. These symptoms of schizophrenia are often emphasized, since they can be dramatic, can erupt suddenly when a patient decompensates into a psychotic episode (often called a psychotic "break," as in break from reality), and are the symptoms most effectively treated by antipsychotic medications. **Delusions** are one type of positive symptom; these usually involve a misinterpretation of perceptions or experiences. The most common content of a delusion in schizophrenia is persecutory, but

TABLE 1-3 Positive symptoms of psychosis and schizophrenia

Delusions
Hallucinations
Distortions or exaggerations in language and communication
Disorganized speech
Disorganized behavior
Catatonic behavior
Agitation

TABLE 1-4 Negative symptoms of schizophrenia

Blunted affect
Emotional withdrawal
Poor rapport
Passivity
Apathetic social withdrawal
Difficulty in abstract thinking
Lack of spontaneity
Stereotyped thinking
Alogia: restrictions in fluency and productivity of thought and speech
Avolition: restrictions in initiation of goal-directed behavior
Anhedonia: lack of pleasure
Attentional impairment

may comprise a variety of other themes including referential (i.e., erroneously thinking that something refers to oneself), somatic, religious, or grandiose. **Hallucinations** are also a type of positive symptom (Table 1-3) and may occur in any sensory modality (e.g., auditory, visual, olfactory, gustatory and tactile), but auditory hallucinations are by far the most common and characteristic hallucinations in schizophrenia. Positive symptoms generally reflect an **excess** of normal functions and, in addition to delusions and hallucinations, may also include distortions or exaggerations in language and communication (disorganized speech) as well as in behavioral monitoring (grossly disorganized or catatonic or agitated behavior).

Negative symptoms are listed in Tables 1-4 and 1-5. Classically, there are at least five types of negative symptoms, all starting with the letter "A" (Table 1-5):

alogia – dysfunction of communication; restrictions in the fluency and productivity of thought and speech

affective blunting or flattening – restrictions in the range and intensity of emotional expression

asociality – reduced social drive and interaction

anhedonia – reduced ability to experience pleasure

avolition – reduced desire, motivation, or persistence; restrictions in the initiation of goal-directed behavior

TABLE 1-5 What are negative symptoms?

Domain	Descriptive Term	Translation
Dysfunction of communication	Alogia	Poverty of speech; e.g., talks little, uses few words
Dysfunction of affect	Blunted affect	Reduced range of emotions (perception, experience and expression); e.g., feels numb or empty inside, recalls few emotional experiences good or bad
Dysfunction of socialization	Asociality	Reduced social drive and interaction; e.g., little sexual interest, few friends, little interest in spending time with (or little time spent with) friends
Dysfunction of capacity for pleasure	Anhedonia	Reduced ability to experience pleasure; e.g., finds previous hobbies or interests unpleasurable
Dysfunction of motivation	Avolition	Reduced desire or motivation persistence; e.g., reduced ability to undertake and complete everyday tasks; may have poor personal hygiene

Negative symptoms in schizophrenia are commonly considered a reduction in normal functions, such as blunted affect, emotional withdrawal, poor rapport, passivity and apathetic social withdrawal, difficulty in abstract thinking, stereotyped thinking and lack of spontaneity. These symptoms are associated with long periods of hospitalization and poor social functioning. Although this reduction in normal functioning may not be as dramatic as positive symptoms, it is interesting to note that negative symptoms of schizophrenia determine whether a patient ultimately functions well or has a poor outcome. Certainly patients will have disruptions in their ability to interact with others when their positive symptoms are out of control, but their degree of negative symptoms will largely determine whether they can live independently, maintain stable social relationships, or reenter the workplace.

Negative symptoms in schizophrenia can be either primary or secondary (Table 1-6). Primary negative symptoms are considered to be those that are core features of the primary deficits of schizophrenia itself. Other deficits of schizophrenia that may manifest themselves as negative symptoms are thought to be secondary to the positive symptoms of psychosis or secondary to EPS (extrapyramidal symptoms) caused by antipsychotic medications. Negative symptoms can also be secondary to depressive symptoms or environmental deprivation. As shown in Table 1-6, there is debate as to whether this distinction of primary from secondary negative symptoms is important.

Since negative symptoms are so important to the outcome of schizophrenia, it is important to measure them in clinical practice (Table 1-7). Although formal rating scales such as those listed in Table 1-8 can be used to measure negative symptoms in research studies, in clinical practice it may be more practical to identify and monitor negative symptoms quickly by observation alone (Figure 1-2) or by some simple questioning (Figure 1-3). A more quantitative assessment for clinical practice can be rapidly made by rating just four items taken from formal rating scales and shown in Table 1-9; namely, reduced range of emotions, reduced interests, reduced social drive, and restricted speech quantity.

Negative symptoms are not just part of the syndrome of schizophrenia – they can also be part of a "prodrome" that begins with subsyndromal symptoms which do not meet the diagnostic criteria of schizophrenia and occur before the onset of the full syndrome (Figure 1-4). Prodromal negative symptoms are important to detect and monitor over time in

TABLE 1-6 Primary and secondary negative symptoms

Primary: Inherent to the disease process itself

Secondary: Result from other factors, such as depression, extrapyramidal symptoms (EPS), suspicious withdrawal

Deficit syndrome: Enduring primary negative symptoms

Is the distinction important?

YES

Secondary can mimic primary negative symptoms

e.g., unresponsive facial expression:

■ Sign of reduced emotional responsiveness and experience, anhedonia?
■ Result of EPS?

NO

Negative symptoms, whether primary or secondary, still impair outcomes and should be avoided

---

TABLE 1-7 Why measure negative symptoms?

1. In clinical trials
   ■ To measure efficacy of interventions in treating negative symptoms
     – pharmacological interventions
     – psychosocial, cognitive, and behavioral interventions
2. In clinical practice
   ■ To identify patients in your practice who have negative symptoms and the severity of these symptoms
   ■ To monitor response of your patients to pharmacological and nonpharmacological interventions

---

TABLE 1-8 Scales used to assess negative symptoms

BPRS	Brief Psychiatric Rating Scale (retardation factor)
PANSS	Positive and Negative Syndrome Scale (negative symptom subscale; negative factor)
SANS	Scale for Assessment of Negative Symptoms
NSA-16	Negative Symptom Assessment
SDS	Schedule for the Deficit Syndrome

---

high-risk patients so that treatment can be initiated at the first signs of psychosis (Figure 1-4). Negative symptoms can also persist between psychotic episodes once schizophrenia has begun and reduce social and occupational functioning in the absence of positive symptoms.

Because of the increasing recognition of the importance of negative symptoms, their detection and treatment are now being emphasized. Despite the fact that our current antipsychotic drug treatments are limited in their ability to treat negative symptoms, psychosocial interventions along with antipsychotics can be helpful in reducing negative symptoms. There is even the possibility that instituting treatment for negative symptoms during the prodromal phase of schizophrenia may delay or prevent the onset of the illness, but this is still a matter of current research.

Beyond positive and negative symptoms of schizophrenia

Although not recognized formally as part of the diagnostic criteria for schizophrenia, numerous studies subcategorize the symptoms of this illness into five dimensions: not

Key Negative Symptoms Identified Solely on Observation

Reduced speech: Patient has restricted speech quantity, uses few words and nonverbal responses. May also have impoverished content of speech, when words convey little meaning*

A

Poor grooming: Patient has poor grooming and hygiene, clothes are dirty or stained, or subject has an odor*

B

Limited eye contact: Patient rarely makes eye contact with the interviewer*

C

*Symptoms described are for patients at the more severe end of the spectrum.

FIGURE 1-2 Negative symptoms identified by observation. Some negative symptoms of schizophrenia – such as reduced speech, poor grooming, and limited eye contact – can be identified solely by observing the patient.

Key Negative Symptoms Identified with Some Questioning

Reduced emotional responsiveness: Patient exhibits few emotions or changes in facial expression and, when questioned, can recall few occasions of emotional experience*

A

Reduced interest: Reduced interests and hobbies, little or nothing stimulates interest, limited life goals and inability to proceed with them*

B

Reduced social drive: Patient has reduced desire to initiate social contacts and may have few or no friends or close relationships*

C

*Symptoms described are for patients at the more severe end of the spectrum.

FIGURE 1-3 Negative symptoms identified by questioning. Other negative symptoms of schizophrenia can be identified by simple questioning. For example, brief questioning can reveal the degree of emotional responsiveness, interest level in hobbies or pursuing life goals, and desire to initiate and maintain social contacts.

TABLE 1-9 Selected items for rapid clinical assessment

1. **Reduced range of emotions**

Base rating on the subject's answers to the following queries:

Have you felt anxious, nervous, or worried during the past week? What has that been like for you? What makes you feel this way? (Repeat for sad, happy, proud, scared, surprised, an angry)

During the last week, were there times when you felt numb or empty inside?

1. Normal range of emotion
2. Minimal reduction in range, may be extreme of normal
3. Range seems restricted relative to a normal person but subject convincingly reports at least four emotions
4. Subject convincingly identifies two or three emotional experiences
5. Subject can convincingly identify only one emotional experience
6. Subject reports little or no emotional range

Reduced range of emotion: Ask the patient whether he or she has experienced a range of emotions in the past week and rate according to the number of emotions described (Note that the ability to experience emotion is different from the ability to display affect)

2. **Reduced interests**

Base rating on assessment of range and intensity of subject's interests

What do you enjoy doing? What else do you enjoy? Have you done these things in past week? Are you interested in what is going on in the world? Do you read the newspapers? Do you watch the news on TV? Can you tell me about some of the important news stories of the past week? Do you like sports? What is your favorite sport? Which is your favorite team? Who are the top players in this sport? Have you played in any sport during the past week?

1. Normal sense of purpose
2. Minimal reduction in purpose, may be extreme of normal
3. Life goals somewhat vague but current activities suggest purpose
4. Subject has difficulty coming up with life goals but activities are directed toward limited goal or goals
5. Goals are very limited or have to be suggested and activities are not focused toward achieving any of them
6. No identifiable life goals

Reduced Interests: Assess whether the patient has a normal range and intensity of interests

3. **Reduced social drive**

Rate based on patient responses to queries:

Do you live alone or with someone else?

Do you like to be around other people? Do you spend much time with others?

Do you have difficulty feeling close to them?

How are your friends? How often do you see them? Did you see them this past week? Have you called them on the phone? When you got together this past week, who decided what to do and where to go?

Is anyone concerned about your happiness and well-being?

1. Normal social drive
2. Minimal reduction in social drive, may be extreme of normal
3. Desire for social interactions seems somewhat reduced
4. Obvious reduction in desire to initiate social contacts, but a number of contacts are initiated each week
5. Marked reduction in the subject's desire to initiate social contacts, but a few contacts are maintained at subject's initiation (as with family)
6. No desire to initiate any social interactions

Reduced social drive: Assess the level of social drive by probing the type of social interactions and their frequency. Remember to rate in reference to an age-matched normal.

(Cont.)

TABLE 1-9 (*Cont.*)

2. **Restricted speech quantity**

No specific question; rate based on observations during the interview.

1. Normal speech quantity
2. Minimal reduction in quantity, may be extreme of normal
3. Speech quantity is reduced, but more obtained with minimal prodding
4. Flow of speech is maintained only by regularly prodding
5. Responses usually limited to a few words and/or detail is only obtained by prodding or bribing
6. Responses usually nonverbal or limited to one or two words despite efforts to elicit more

Restricted speech quantity: This item requires no specific questions and is rated based on observing the patient's speech during the interview.

All ratings should assess the function/behavior of the patient in reference to a normal age-matched person.

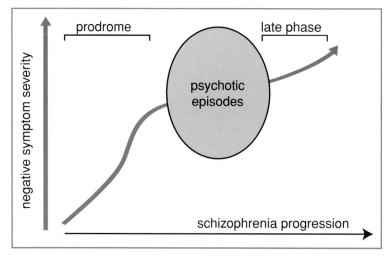

FIGURE 1-4 Negative symptoms in the prodromal phase. Negative symptoms of schizophrenia may occur during the prodromal phase, prior to developing the full syndrome of schizophrenia with both positive and negative symptoms. Theoretically, if such prodromal negative symptoms could be identified early and treated with psychosocial or pharmacological interventions prior to the onset of a psychotic break, it might be possible to delay or even prevent the onset of full-syndrome schizophrenia.

just positive and negative symptoms but also cognitive symptoms, aggressive symptoms, and affective symptoms (Figure 1-5). This is perhaps a more sophisticated if complicated manner of describing the symptoms of schizophrenia.

The overlaps among these five symptom dimensions are shown in Figure 1-6A, and some potentially overlapping symptoms are shown in Figure 1-6B. That is, aggressive symptoms such as assaultiveness, verbally abusive behaviors, and frank violence can occur with positive symptoms such as delusions and hallucinations, yet this is not always the case. It can be difficult to separate the symptoms of formal cognitive dysfunction and those of affective dysfunction from negative symptoms, as shown in Figure 1-6B. Since research is attempting to localize the specific areas of brain dysfunction for each of these

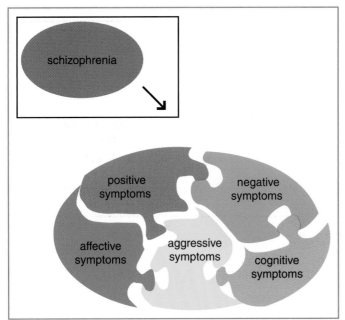

FIGURE 1-5 Five symptom dimensions of schizophrenia. The syndrome of schizophrenia can be conceptualized as consisting of five symptom dimensions rather than just the two dimensions of positive and negative symptoms shown in Figure 1-1. This deconstruction of the schizophrenia syndrome thus includes not only positive symptoms and negative symptoms but also cognitive, affective, and aggressive symptoms.

symptom domains and scientists are also attempting to develop better treatments for the often neglected negative, cognitive, and affective symptoms of schizophrenia, there are ongoing attempts to try to quantify and measure such symptoms independently.

In particular, neuropsychological assessment batteries are being developed to quantitate cognitive symptoms, to show how they are independent of the other symptoms of schizophrenia, and to detect cognitive improvement after treatment with a number of novel psychotropic drugs currently being tested. Cognitive symptoms of schizophrenia and other illnesses where psychosis may be an associated feature can overlap with negative symptoms, so test batteries attempt to parse cognitive symptoms from negative symptoms. Overlapping symptoms can include the thought disorder of schizophrenia and the sometimes odd use of language, including incoherence, loose associations, and neologisms. Impaired attention and impaired information processing are other specific cognitive impairments associated with schizophrenia. In fact, the most common and severe of the cognitive impairments in schizophrenia can include impaired verbal fluency (ability to produce spontaneous speech), problems with serial learning (of a list of items or a sequence of events), and impairment in vigilance for executive functioning (problems with sustaining and focusing attention, concentrating, prioritizing, and modulating behavior based on social cues).

Important cognitive symptoms of schizophrenia are listed in Table 1-10. These do not include symptoms of dementia and memory disturbance more characteristic of Alzheimer's disease, but cognitive symptoms of schizophrenia emphasize "executive dysfunction," which includes problems in representing and maintaining goals, allocating attentional resources, evaluating and monitoring performance, and utilizing these skills to solve problems. It is important to recognize and monitor cognitive symptoms of schizophrenia because they are the single strongest correlate of real-world functioning – even stronger than negative symptoms.

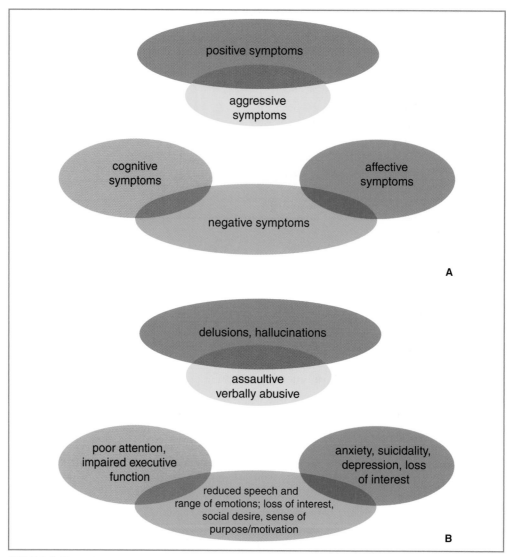

FIGURE 1-6A and B Symptom overlap. Although schizophrenia may be conceptually divided into five symptom dimensions, as shown in Figure 1-5, in reality there is a good deal of overlap among these separate symptom dimensions (**A**). In particular, aggressive symptoms such as assaultiveness and verbal abuse frequently occur in association with positive symptoms (**B**). Impairment in attention and executive functioning as well as affective symptoms such as loss of interest may be difficult to distinguish from negative symptoms (**B**).

Symptoms of schizophrenia are not necessarily unique to schizophrenia

It is important to recognize that several illnesses other than schizophrenia can share some of the same five symptom dimensions described here for schizophrenia and shown in Figure 1-5. Thus, disorders in addition to schizophrenia that can have **positive symptoms** include bipolar disorder, schizoaffective disorder, psychotic depression, Alzheimer's disease and other organic dementias, childhood psychotic illnesses, drug-induced psychoses, and others (Figure 1-7).

Negative symptoms can also occur in other disorders and can also overlap with cognitive and affective symptoms occurring in these disorders. However, as a primary deficit

TABLE 1-10 Cognitive symptoms of schizophrenia

Problems representing and maintaining goals
Problems allocating attentional resources
Problems focusing attention
Problems sustaining attention
Problems evaluating functions
Problems monitoring performance
Problems prioritizing
Problems modulating behavior based upon social cues
Problems with serial learning
Impaired verbal fluency
Difficulty with problem solving

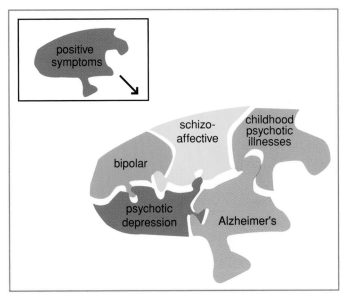

FIGURE 1-7 Positive symptoms across disorders. Positive symptoms are not associated only with schizophrenia but can also occur in several other disorders that may be associated with psychotic symptoms, including bipolar disorder, schizoaffective disorder, childhood psychotic illnesses, Alzheimer's disease and other organic dementias, psychotic depression, and others.

state (Figure 1-8), negative symptoms are unique to schizophrenia. On the other hand, negative symptoms that are secondary to other causes are common in schizophrenia but not necessarily unique to this disorder (Figure 1-8).

Schizophrenia is certainly not the only disorder with **cognitive symptoms**. Autism, poststroke (vascular or multi-infarct) dementia, Alzheimer's disease, and many other organic dementias (parkinsonian/Lewy-body dementia; Pick's disease or frontotemporal lobar degeneration, etc.) can also be associated with cognitive dysfunctions similar to those seen in schizophrenia (Figure 1-9).

Finally, **aggressive and hostile symptoms** occur in numerous other disorders, especially those with problems of impulse control. Symptoms include overt hostility, such as verbal or physical abusiveness or even assault; self-injurious behaviors including suicide; and arson or other property damage. Other types of impulsiveness, such as sexual acting out, are also in this category of aggressive and hostile symptoms. These same symptoms are frequently associated with bipolar disorder, childhood psychosis, borderline personality disorder, antisocial

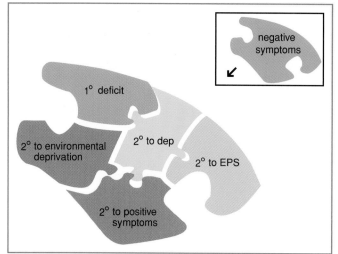

FIGURE 1-8 Causes of negative symptoms. Negative symptoms in schizophrenia can either be a primary core deficit of the illness (1° deficit), or secondary to depression (2° to dep), secondary to extrapyramidal symptoms (2° to EPS), secondary to environmental deprivation, or even secondary to positive symptoms in schizophrenia.

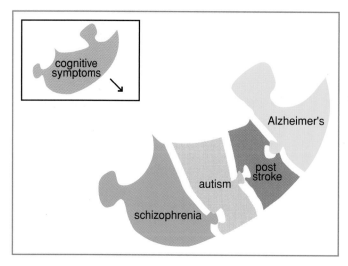

FIGURE 1-9 Cognitive symptoms across disorders. Cognitive symptoms are not associated only with schizophrenia but also with several other disorders including autism, Alzheimer's disease, following cerebrovascular accidents (poststroke) and many others.

personality disorder, drug abuse, Alzheimer's and other dementias, attention deficit hyperactivity disorder, conduct disorders in children, and many others (Figure 1-10).

Affective symptoms are frequently associated with schizophrenia, but this does not necessarily mean that they fulfill the diagnostic criteria for a comorbid anxiety or affective disorder. Nevertheless, depressed mood, anxious mood, guilt, tension, irritability, and worry frequently accompany schizophrenia. These various symptoms are also prominent features of major depressive disorder, psychotic depression, bipolar disorder, schizoaffective disorder, organic dementias, childhood psychotic disorders, and treatment-resistant cases of depression, bipolar disorder, and schizophrenia, among others (Figure 1-11).

Brain circuits and symptom dimensions in schizophrenia

Just as is the case for other psychiatric disorders, the various symptoms of schizophrenia are hypothesized to be localized in unique brain regions (Figure 1-12). Specifically, the positive

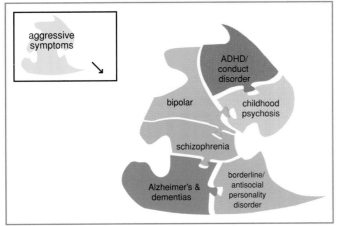

FIGURE 1-10 Aggressive symptoms across disorders. Aggressive symptoms and hostility are associated with several conditions in addition to schizophrenia, including bipolar disorder, attention deficit hyperactivity disorder (ADHD), conduct disorder, childhood psychosis, borderline personality disorder and antisocial personality disorder, Alzheimer's disease, and other dementias.

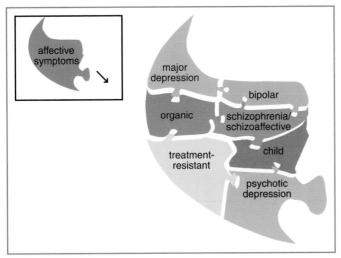

FIGURE 1-11 Affective symptoms across disorders. Affective symptoms are a hallmark not only of major depressive disorder but are also frequently associated with other psychiatric disorders, including bipolar disorder, schizophrenia and schizoaffective disorder, childhood mood disorders, psychotic forms of depression, treatment-resistant mood and psychotic disorders, and organic causes of depression such as substance abuse.

symptoms of schizophrenia have long been hypothesized to be localized to malfunctioning mesolimbic circuits, especially involving the nucleus accumbens. The nucleus accumbens is considered to be part of the brain's reward circuitry, so it is not surprising that problems with reward and motivation in schizophrenia – symptoms that can overlap with negative symptoms and lead to smoking, drug and alcohol abuse – may be linked to this brain area as well.

The prefrontal cortex is considered to be a key node in the nexus of malfunctioning cerebral circuitry responsible for each of the remaining symptoms of schizophrenia: specifically, the mesocortical and ventromedial prefrontal cortex with negative symptoms and affective symptoms, the dorsolateral prefrontal cortex with cognitive symptoms, and the orbitofrontal cortex and its connections to the amygdala with aggressive, impulsive symptoms (Figure 1-12).

This model is obviously oversimplified and reductionistic, because every brain area has several functions and every function is certainly distributed to more than more brain area.

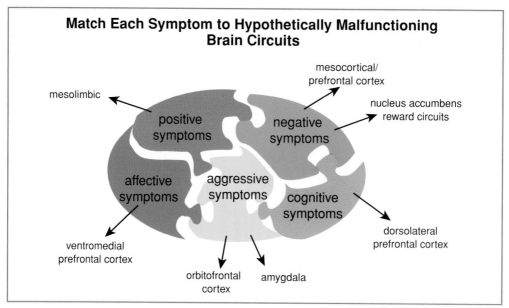

Match Each Symptom to Hypothetically Malfunctioning Brain Circuits

FIGURE 1-12 Localization of symptom domains. The different symptom domains of schizophrenia are hypothesized to be regulated by unique brain regions. **Positive symptoms** of schizophrenia are hypothetically modulated by malfunctioning mesolimbic circuits, while **negative symptoms** are hypothetically linked to malfunctioning mesocortical circuits and may also involve mesolimbic regions such as the nucleus accumbens, which is part of the brain's reward circuitry and thus plays a role in motivation. The nucleus accumbens may also be involved in the increased rate of substance use and abuse seen in patients with schizophrenia. **Affective symptoms** are associated with the ventromedial prefrontal cortex, while **aggressive symptoms** (related to impulse control) are associated with abnormal information processing in orbitofrontal cortex and amygdala, whereas **cognitive symptoms** are associated with problematic information processing in dorsolateral prefrontal cortex. Although there is overlap in function among different brain regions, understanding which brain regions may be predominantly involved in specific symptoms can aid in customization of treatment to the particular symptom profile of each individual patient with schizophrenia.

Nevertheless, allocating specific symptom dimensions to unique brain areas not only assists research studies but has both heuristic and clinical value. Specifically, every patient has unique symptoms and unique responses to medication. In order to optimize and individualize treatment, it can be useful to consider which specific symptoms any given patient is expressing and therefore which areas of that particular patient's brain are hypothetically malfunctioning (Figure 1-12). Each brain area has unique neurotransmitters, receptors, enzymes, and genes that regulate it, with some overlap but also with some unique regional differences; knowing this can help the clinician in choosing medications and monitoring the effectiveness of treatment.

For example, positive symptoms of schizophrenia are theoretically most robustly linked to the mesolimbic/nucleus accumbens brain area and to the neurotransmitter dopamine, with perhaps secondary involvement of the neurotransmitters serotonin, glutamate, gamma-aminobutyric acid (GABA), and others (Figure 1-13). On the other hand, emotional symptoms such as affective and social symptoms are more robustly linked to orbital, medial, and ventral areas of the prefrontal cortex, with executive cognitive symptoms related to the dorsolateral prefrontal cortex (Figure 1-14). Neurotransmitters and key regulatory molecules for the dorsolateral prefrontal cortex include not only dopamine but also several others (Figure 1-15).

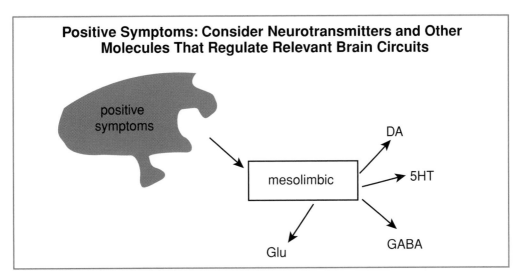

Positive Symptoms: Consider Neurotransmitters and Other Molecules That Regulate Relevant Brain Circuits

positive symptoms

mesolimbic

DA

5HT

Glu

GABA

FIGURE 1-13 **Positive symptoms and mesolimbic circuits.** Positive symptoms of schizophrenia are associated with malfunctioning mesolimbic circuits; the neurotransmitters that regulate mesolimbic neuronal functioning include dopamine (DA), which plays a predominant regulatory role, as well as several other neurotransmitters that play important but perhaps lesser regulatory roles, such as serotonin (5HT), gamma-aminobutyric acid (GABA), and glutamate (glu).

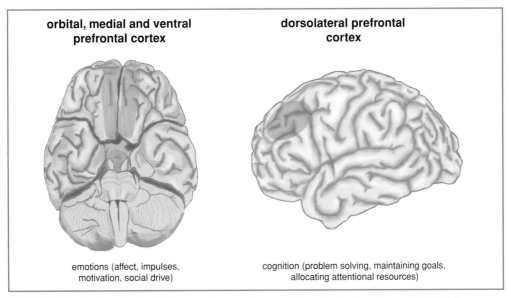

orbital, medial and ventral prefrontal cortex

dorsolateral prefrontal cortex

emotions (affect, impulses, motivation, social drive)

cognition (problem solving, maintaining goals, allocating attentional resources)

FIGURE 1-14 **Emotional and cognitive symptoms and mesocortical circuits.** Emotional symptoms of schizophrenia (such as affective symptoms, impulsive symptoms, absence of motivation, absence of social drive) are theoretically mediated by different regions of the prefrontal cortex than are cognitive symptoms. Specifically, emotional symptoms of schizophrenia are hypothetically associated with abnormal information processing in the orbital, medial, and ventral prefrontal cortex (left), while cognitive symptoms of schizophrenia are hypothetically associated with abnormal information processing in the dorsolateral prefrontal cortex (right).

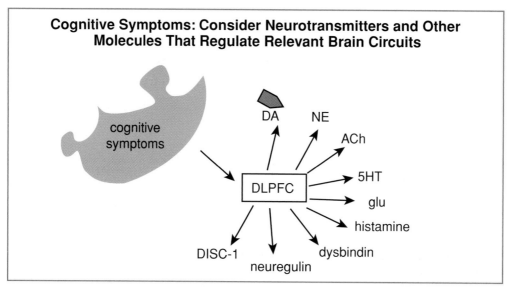

Cognitive Symptoms: Consider Neurotransmitters and Other Molecules That Regulate Relevant Brain Circuits

FIGURE 1-15 **Cognitive symptoms and dorsolateral prefrontal cortex.** The dorsolateral prefrontal cortex, which is linked to cognitive symptoms of schizophrenia, is modulated by the neurotransmitter dopamine (DA) as well as by several other neurotransmitters, including norepinephrine (NE), acetylcholine (ACh), serotonin (5HT), glutamate (glu), and histamine (HA). Circuits in prefrontal cortex are also modulated by numerous molecules important in synapse formation such as dysbindin, neuregulin, and DISC-1 (disrupted in schizophrenia-1).

What is the point of deconstructing the diagnosis of schizophrenia into its symptom domains and then matching each symptom to a hypothetically malfunctioning brain circuit and the neurotransmitters that regulate that brain area? This strategy not only helps the clinician to develop a unique profile of symptoms to target in each individual patient but also provides a specifically tailored set of psychopharmacological treatment tactics for each individual. That is, each neurotransmitter regulating a given circuit is associated with unique pharmacological agents that either boost or block it, depending on the outcome desired (Figure 1-16). When one agent for a given neurotransmitter is ineffective, this approach suggests not only another agent for that same neurotransmitter but also agents for other neurotransmitters that may work together to form a logical set of cotherapies to relieve symptoms. An additional bonus to this approach is that it also suggests which specific genes may be involved in any given symptom in any given brain area (Figure 1-17). This latter information will be critical for developing rational genetic approaches to risk assessment for individual patients and their families and will help in interpreting the results of functional neuroimaging tests to assess these patients' biological endophenotypes, indicating how efficient their information processing is in specific brain regions and whether they are enhancing their chances of symptom relief and reducing their chances of relapse.

Neurotransmitters and circuits in schizophrenia

Dopamine

The biological basis of schizophrenia remains unknown. However, the monoamine neurotransmitter dopamine (DA) has long played a prominent role in the hypotheses of

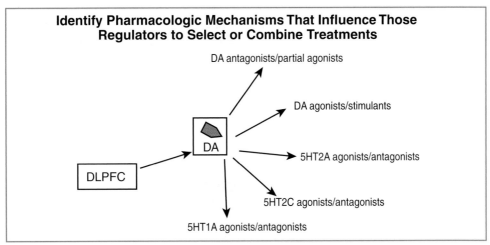

FIGURE 1-16 Pharmacological mechanisms influencing dopamine. By matching individual symptoms to a particular brain region and the neurotransmitters that regulate it, clinicians can identify pharmacological mechanisms that influence those regulators. This information can then be utilized to select specific drugs acting on desired pharmacological mechanisms to target the relief of specific symptoms. Theoretically, this occurs by drugs acting on neurotransmitters to change the efficiency of information processing in specific brain areas with hypothetically malfunctioning circuitry. For example, as shown in Figure 1-15, the dorsolateral prefrontal cortex (DLPFC) is regulated by dopamine (DA) and serotonin (5HT). Thus, agents that act on DA and/or serotonin, such as agonists or antagonists of dopamine at D1 and D2 receptors, as well as agonists and antagonists of serotonin at 5HT2A, 5HT2C, and 5HT1A receptors, may all affect information processing in this brain area and thus, cognitive function.

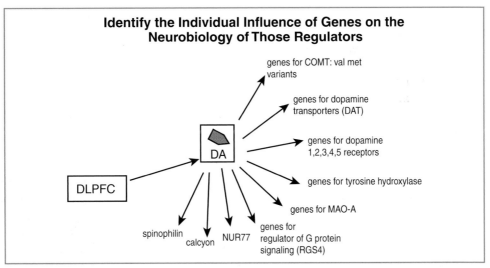

FIGURE 1-17 Genes influencing dopamine. Determining the brain regions and regulatory neurotransmitters involved in specific symptoms of schizophrenia aids in the identification of genes that may be involved in the manifestation of those symptoms. For example, dopamine (DA) neurotransmission, which modulates activity in the dorsolateral prefrontal cortex (DLPFC), is influenced by several genes including genes for catechol-O-methyl-transferase (COMT), genes for the dopamine transporter (DAT), genes for various dopamine receptors, and many other genes, several of which are shown here. Identifying genetic contributions to symptoms of schizophrenia may ultimately allow for genetic approaches to risk assessment for patients and their families as well as assist in the design of more effective psychopharmacological agents for treating the symptoms of schizophrenia.

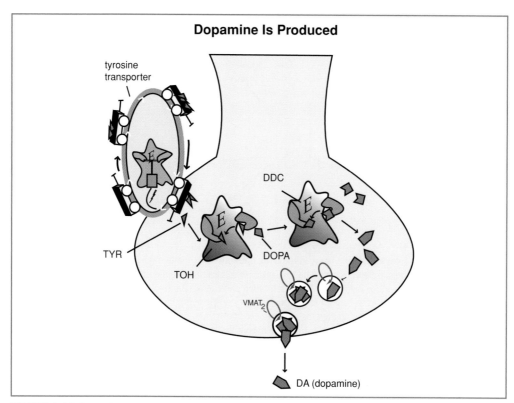

Dopamine Is Produced

FIGURE 1-18 Dopamine synthesis. Tyrosine, a precursor to dopamine, is taken up into dopamine nerve terminals via a tyrosine transporter and converted into DOPA by the enzyme tyrosine hydroxylase (TOH). DOPA is then converted into dopamine (DA) by the enzyme DOPA decarboxylase (DDC). After synthesis, dopamine is packaged into synaptic vesicles via the vesicular monoamine transporter (VMAT2) and stored there until its release into the synapse during neurotransmission.

schizophrenia. To understand the potential role of dopamine in schizophrenia, it is first important to review how dopamine is synthesized, metabolized, and regulated; the role of dopamine receptors; and the localization of key dopamine pathways in the brain.

Dopaminergic neurons

Dopaminergic neurons utilize the neurotransmitter DA, which is synthesized in dopaminergic nerve terminals from the amino acid tyrosine after it is taken up into the neuron from the extracellular space and bloodstream by a tyrosine pump, or transporter (Figure 1-18). Tyrosine is converted into DA first by the rate-limiting enzyme tyrosine hydroxylase (TOH) and then by the enzyme dopa decarboxylase (DDC) (Figure 1-18). DA is then taken up into synaptic vesicles by a vesicular monoamine transporter (VMAT2) and stored there until it is used during neurotransmission.

The DA neuron has a presynaptic transporter (reuptake pump) called DAT, which is unique for DA and which terminates DA's synaptic action by whisking it out of the synapse back into the presynaptic nerve terminal, where it can be re-stored in synaptic vesicles for subsequent reuse in another neurotransmission (Figure 1-19). DATs are not found in high density at the axon terminals of all DA neurons, however. For example, in prefrontal cortex, DATs are relatively sparse, and DA is inactivated by other mechanisms. Excess DA that

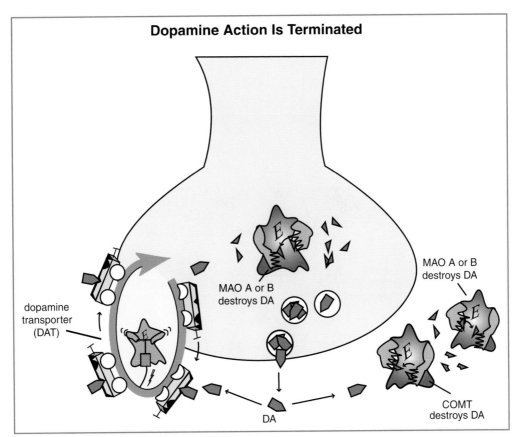

Dopamine Action Is Terminated

MAO A or B destroys DA

dopamine transporter (DAT)

MAO A or B destroys DA

DA

COMT destroys DA

FIGURE 1-19 Dopamine's action is terminated. Dopamine's action can be terminated through multiple mechanisms. Dopamine can be transported out of the synaptic cleft and back into the presynaptic neuron via the dopamine transporter (DAT), where it may be repackaged for future use. Alternatively, dopamine may be broken down extracellularly via the enzyme catechol-O-methyltransferase (COMT). Other enzymes that break down dopamine are monoamine oxidase A (MAO-A) and monoamine oxidase B (MAO-B), which are present in mitochondria within the presynaptic neuron and in other cells such as glia.

escapes storage in synaptic vesicles can be destroyed within the neuron by the enzymes monoamine oxidase (MAO) A or MAO-B or outside the neuron by the enzyme catechol-O-methyl transferase (COMT) (Figure 1-19). DA that diffuses away from synapses can also be transported by norepinephrine transporters (NETs) as a "false" substrate, and DA action will be terminated in this manner.

Receptors for dopamine also regulate dopaminergic neurotransmission (Figure 1-20). The DA transporter DAT and the vesicular transporter VMAT2 are both types of receptors. A plethora of additional dopamine receptors exist, including at least five pharmacological subtypes and several more molecular isoforms. Perhaps the most extensively investigated dopamine receptor is the dopamine-2 receptor, as it is stimulated by dopamine agonists for the treatment of Parkinson's disease and blocked by dopamine antagonist antipsychotics for the treatment of schizophrenia. As will be discussed in greater detail in Chapter 2, dopamine 1, 2, 3, and 4 receptors are all blocked by some atypical antipsychotic drugs, but it is not clear to what extent dopamine 1, 3, or 4 receptors contribute to the clinical properties of these drugs.

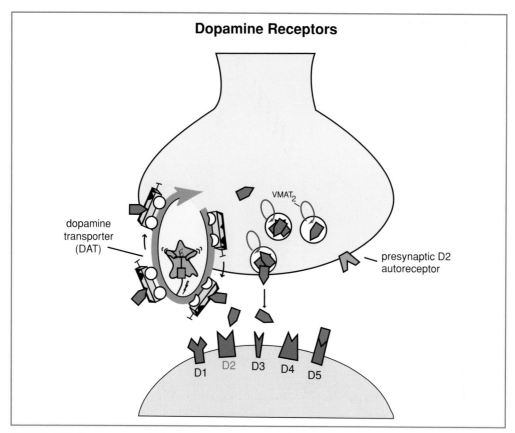

FIGURE 1-20 Dopamine receptors. Shown here are receptors for dopamine that regulate its neurotransmission. The dopamine transporter (DAT) exists presynaptically and is responsible for clearing excess dopamine out of the synapse. The vesicular monoamine transporter (VMAT2) takes dopamine up into synaptic vesicles for future neurotransmission. There is also a presynaptic dopamine-2 autoreceptor, which regulates release of dopamine from the presynaptic neuron. In addition, there are several postsynaptic receptors. These include dopamine-1, dopamine-2, dopamine-3, dopamine-4, and dopamine-5 receptors. The functions of the dopamine-2 receptors are best understood, because this is the primary binding site for virtually all antipsychotic agents as well as for dopamine agonists used to treat Parkinson's disease.

Dopamine D2 receptors can be presynaptic, where they function as autoreceptors (Figure 1-20). Presynaptic D2 receptors thus act as "gatekeepers," either allowing DA release when they are not occupied by DA (Figure 1-21A) or inhibiting DA release when DA builds up in the synapse and occupies the gatekeeping presynaptic autoreceptor (Figure 1-21B). Such receptors are located either on the axon terminal (Figure 1-22) or on the other end of the neuron in the somatodendritic area (Figure 1-23). In both cases, occupancy of these D2 receptors provides negative feedback input, or a braking action on the release of dopamine from the presynaptic neuron.

Key dopamine pathways in the brain

Four well-defined dopamine pathways in the brain plus a newly discovered fifth pathway for dopamine are shown in Figure 1-24. They include the mesolimbic, mesocortical, nigrostriatal, and tuberoinfundibular dopamine DA pathways. The new pathway innervates the thalamus.

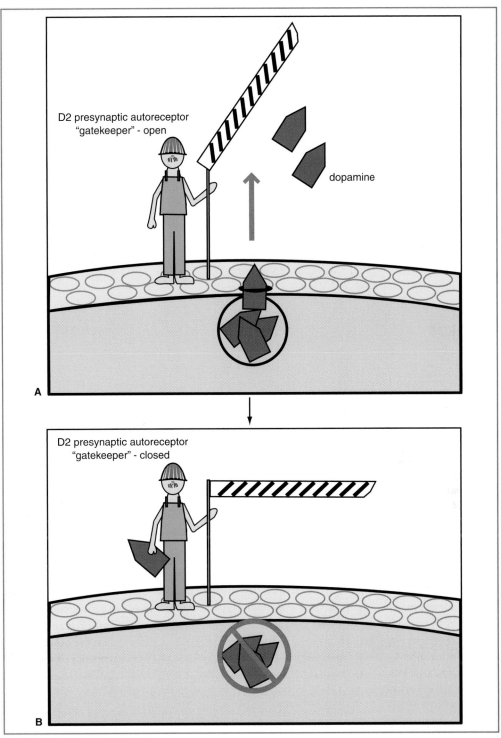

FIGURE 1-21A and B Presynaptic dopamine-2 autoreceptors. Presynaptic dopamine-2 autoreceptors are "gatekeepers" for dopamine. That is, when these gatekeeping receptors are not bound by dopamine (no dopamine in the gatekeeper's hand), they open a molecular gate, allowing dopamine release (**A**). However, when dopamine binds to the gatekeeping receptors (now the gatekeeper has dopamine in his hand), they close the molecular gate and prevent dopamine from being released (**B**).

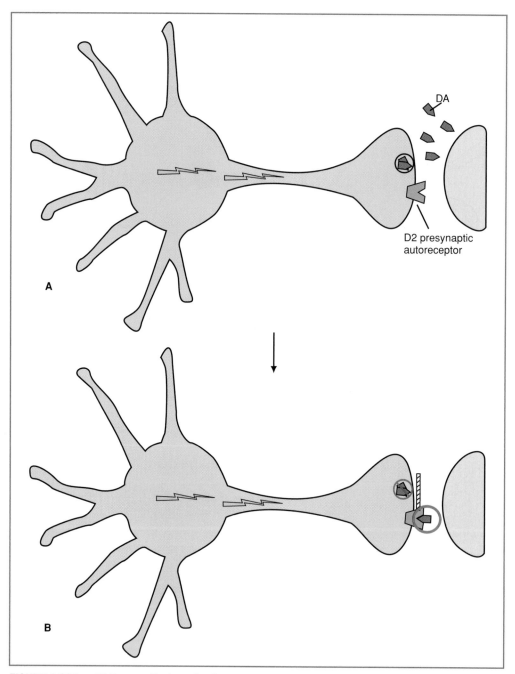

FIGURE 1-22A and B Presynaptic dopamine-2 autoreceptors. Presynaptic dopamine-2 autoreceptors can be located on the axon terminal, as shown here. When dopamine builds up in the synapse (**A**), it is available to bind to the autoreceptor, which then inhibits dopamine release (**B**).

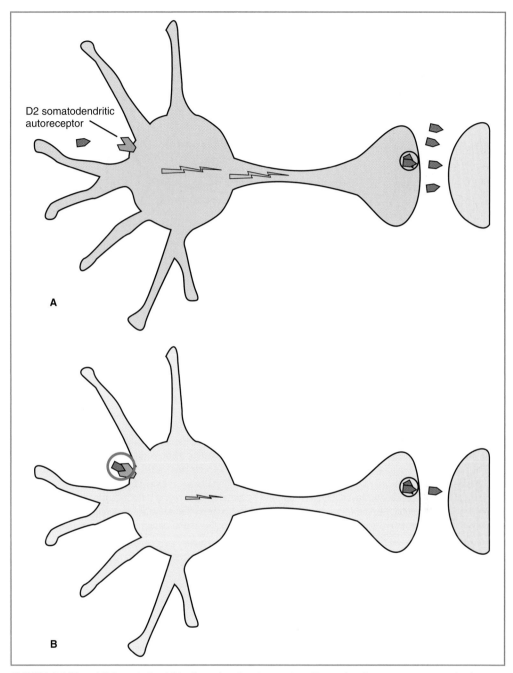

FIGURE 1-23A and B Somatodendritic dopamine-2 autoreceptors. Dopamine-2 autoreceptors can also be located in the somatodendritic area, as shown here (**A**). When dopamine binds to the receptor here, it shuts off neuronal impulse flow in the dopamine neuron (see loss of lightning bolts in the neuron in **B**), and this stops further dopamine release.

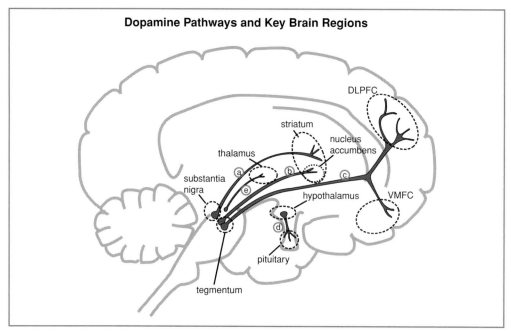

Dopamine Pathways and Key Brain Regions

FIGURE 1-24 Five dopamine pathways in the brain. The neuroanatomy of dopamine neuronal pathways in the brain can explain the symptoms of schizophrenia as well as the therapeutic effects and side effects of antipsychotic drugs. (a) The **nigrostriatal dopamine pathway**, which projects from the substantia nigra to the basal ganglia or striatum, is part of the extrapyramidal nervous system and controls motor function and movement. (b) The **mesolimbic dopamine pathway** projects from the midbrain ventral tegmental area to the nucleus accumbens, a part of the limbic system of the brain thought to be involved in many behaviors such as pleasurable sensations, the powerful euphoria of drugs of abuse, as well as delusions and hallucinations of psychosis. (c) A pathway related to the mesolimbic dopamine pathway is the **mesocortical dopamine pathway**. It also projects from the midbrain ventral tegmental area but sends its axons to areas of the prefrontal cortex, where they may have a role in mediating cognitive symptoms (dorsolateral prefrontal cortex) and affective symptoms (ventromedial prefrontal cortex) of schizophrenia. (d) The fourth dopamine pathway of interest, the **tuberoinfundibular dopamine pathway**, projects from the hypothalamus to the anterior pituitary gland and controls prolactin secretion. (e) The fifth dopamine pathway arises from multiple sites, including the periaqueductal gray, ventral mesencephalon, hypothalamic nuclei, and lateral parabrachial nucleus, and it projects to the thalamus. Its function is not currently well known.

Mesolimbic dopamine pathway and the mesolimbic dopamine hypothesis of positive symptoms of schizophrenia

The **mesolimbic dopamine pathway** projects from dopaminergic cell bodies in the ventral tegmental area of the brainstem to axon terminals in one of the limbic areas of the brain, namely the nucleus accumbens in the ventral striatum (Figure 1-24). This pathway is thought to have an important role in several emotional behaviors, including the positive symptoms of psychosis, such as delusions and hallucinations (Figure 1-25). The mesolimbic dopamine pathway is also important for motivation, pleasure, and reward.

For more than 30 years, it has been observed that diseases or drugs that increase dopamine will enhance or produce positive psychotic symptoms, whereas drugs that decrease dopamine will decrease or stop positive symptoms. For example, stimulant drugs such as amphetamine and cocaine release dopamine and, if given repetitively, can cause a paranoid psychosis virtually indistinguishable from the positive symptoms of schizophrenia.

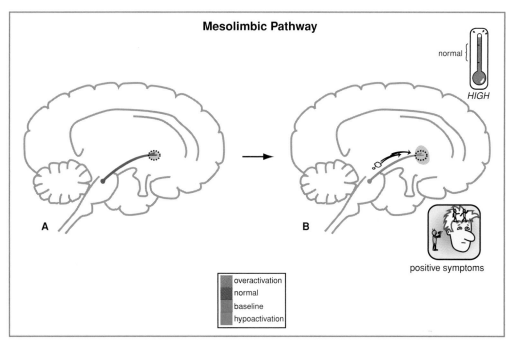

FIGURE 1-25A and B Mesolimbic dopamine pathway. The mesolimbic dopamine pathway, which projects from the ventral tegmental area in the brainstem to the nucleus accumbens in the ventral striatum (**A**), is involved in regulation of emotional behaviors and is believed to be the predominant pathway regulating positive symptoms of psychosis. Specifically, hyperactivity of this pathway is believed to account for delusions and hallucinations (**B**).

All known antipsychotic drugs capable of treating positive psychotic symptoms are blockers of the D2 dopamine receptor. Antipsychotic drugs are discussed in Chapter 2. These observations have been formulated into a theory of psychosis sometimes referred to as the "dopamine hypothesis of schizophrenia." Perhaps a more precise modern designation is the "mesolimbic dopamine hypothesis of positive symptoms of schizophrenia," since it is believed that it is hyperactivity specifically in this particular dopamine pathway that mediates the positive symptoms of psychosis (Figure 1-25 and 1-26). Hyperactivity of the mesolimbic dopamine pathway hypothetically accounts for positive psychotic symptoms, whether those symptoms are part of the illness of schizophrenia or of drug-induced psychosis or whether positive psychotic symptoms accompany mania, depression, or dementia. Hyperactivity of mesolimbic dopamine neurons may also play a role in aggressive and hostile symptoms in schizophrenia and related illnesses, especially if serotonergic control of dopamine is aberrant in patients who lack impulse control.

Mesocortical dopamine pathways and the mesocortical dopamine hypothesis of cognitive, negative, and affective symptoms of schizophrenia

Another pathway also arising from cell bodies in the ventral tegmental area but projecting to areas of the prefrontal cortex is known as the **mesocortical dopamine pathway** (Figures 1-27 and 1-28). Branches of this pathway into the dorsolateral prefrontal cortex are hypothesized to regulate cognition and executive functions (Figure 1-27), whereas its branches into the

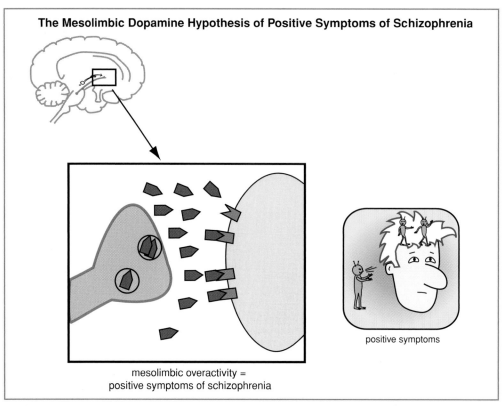

The Mesolimbic Dopamine Hypothesis of Positive Symptoms of Schizophrenia

mesolimbic overactivity =
positive symptoms of schizophrenia

positive symptoms

FIGURE 1-26 Mesolimbic dopamine hypothesis. Hyperactivity of dopamine neurons in the mesolimbic dopamine pathway theoretically mediates the positive symptoms of psychosis such as delusions and hallucinations. This pathway is also involved in pleasure, reward, and reinforcing behavior, and many drugs of abuse interact here.

ventromedial parts of prefrontal cortex are hypothesized to regulate emotions and affect (Figure 1-28). The exact role of the mesocortical dopamine pathway in mediating symptoms of schizophrenia is still a matter of debate, but many researchers believe that cognitive and some negative symptoms of schizophrenia may be due to a **deficit** of dopamine activity in mesocortical projections to dorsolateral prefrontal cortex (Figure 1-27), whereas affective and other negative symptoms of schizophrenia may be due to a **deficit** of dopamine activity in mesocortical projections to ventromedial prefrontal cortex (Figure 1-28).

The behavioral deficit state suggested by negative symptoms certainly implies under-activity or even "burnout" of neuronal systems. This may be related to the consequences of prior excitotoxic overactivity of **glutamate systems** (discussed below). An ongoing degenerative process in the mesocortical dopamine pathway could explain a progressive worsening of symptoms and an ever-increasing deficit state in some schizophrenic patients. This deficit of dopamine in mesocortical projections could also be the consequences of neurodevelopmental abnormalities in the N-methyl-d-aspartate (NMDA) glutamate system, described in the next section. Whatever the cause, a corollary to the original DA hypothesis of schizophrenia now incorporates theories for the cognitive, negative, and affective symptoms and might be more precisely designated as the "mesocortical dopamine hypothesis of cognitive, negative, and affective symptoms of schizophrenia" since it is believed that underactivity specifically in

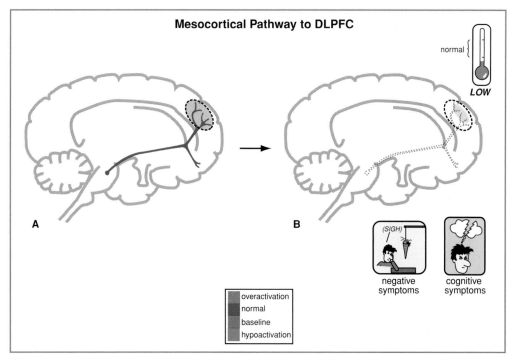

FIGURE 1-27A and B Mesocortical pathway to dorsolateral prefrontal cortex. Another major dopaminergic pathway is the mesocortical dopamine pathway, which projects from the ventral tegmental area to the prefrontal cortex (**A**). Projections specifically to the dorsolateral prefrontal cortex (DLPFC) are believed to be involved in the negative and cognitive symptoms of schizophrenia. In this case, expression of these symptoms is thought to be associated with *hypo*activity of this pathway (**B**).

mesocortical projections to prefrontal cortex mediates the cognitive, negative, and affective symptoms of schizophrenia (Figure 1-29).

Theoretically, increasing dopamine in the mesocortical dopamine pathway might improve the negative, cognitive, and affective symptoms of schizophrenia. However, since there is hypothetically an excess of dopamine elsewhere in the brain within the mesolimbic dopamine pathway, any further increase of dopamine in that pathway would actually worsen positive symptoms. Thus, this state of affairs for dopamine activity in the brain of schizophrenic patients poses a therapeutic dilemma: how do you increase dopamine in the mesocortical pathway while, at the same time, also decreasing dopamine activity in the mesolimbic dopamine pathway? The extent to which atypical antipsychotic medications have provided a solution to this therapeutic dilemma will be discussed in Chapter 2.

Mesolimbic dopamine pathway, reward, and negative symptoms

Dopamine function in schizophrenia may be more complicated than just "too high" in mesolimbic areas and "too low" in mesocortical areas. Instead, it may be that dopamine neurons are better characterized as "out of tune" or "chaotic." A similar phenomenon may be occurring in the mesolimbic dopamine system, with one subset of mesolimbic dopamine neurons out of tune and hyperactive, mediating positive symptoms, and another set of mesolimbic dopamine neurons out of tune but hypoactive, mediating some negative symptoms and malfunctioning reward mechanisms.

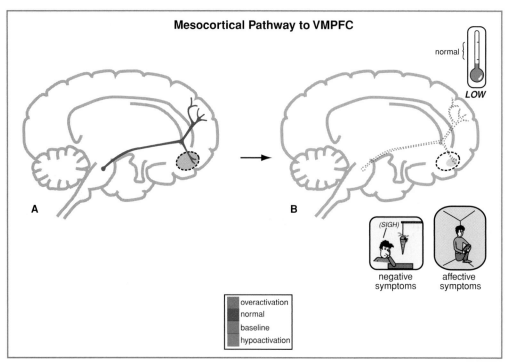

FIGURE 1-28A and B Mesocortical pathway to ventromedial prefrontal cortex. Mesocortical dopamine projections specifically to the ventromedial prefrontal cortex (VMPFC) are believed to mediate negative and affective symptoms associated with schizophrenia (**A**). These symptoms are believed to arise from hypoactivity in this pathway (**B**).

The mesolimbic dopamine pathway is not only the postulated site for the positive symptoms of psychosis but is also thought to be the site of the brain's reward system or pleasure center. When a patient with schizophrenia loses motivation and interest and has anhedonia and lack of pleasure, such symptoms could also implicate a deficient functioning of the mesolimbic dopamine pathway, not just deficient functioning in the mesocortical dopamine pathway.

This idea is further supported by observations that patients treated with antipsychotics, particularly the conventional antipsychotics, can produce a worsening of negative symptoms and a state of "neurolepsis" that looks very much like negative symptoms of schizophrenia. Since the prefrontal cortex does not have a high density of D2 receptors, this implicates possible deficient functioning within the mesolimbic dopamine system, causing inadequate reward mechanisms exhibited as behaviors such as anhedonia and drug abuse as well as negative symptoms exhibited as lack of rewarding social interactions and lack of general motivation and interest. Perhaps the much higher incidence of substance abuse in schizophrenia than in normal adults, especially of nicotine but also of stimulants and other substances of abuse, could be partially explained as an attempt to boost the function of defective mesolimbic dopaminergic pleasure centers, possibly at the cost of activating positive symptoms.

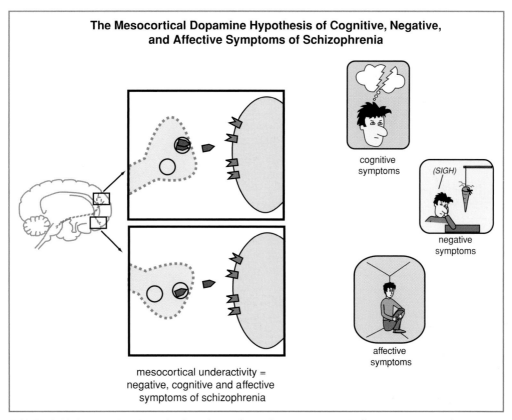

The Mesocortical Dopamine Hypothesis of Cognitive, Negative, and Affective Symptoms of Schizophrenia

cognitive symptoms

negative symptoms

affective symptoms

mesocortical underactivity =
negative, cognitive and affective
symptoms of schizophrenia

FIGURE 1-29 Mesocortical dopamine hypothesis of negative, cognitive, and affective symptoms of schizophrenia. Hypoactivity of dopamine neurons in the mesocortical dopamine pathway theoretically mediates the cognitive, negative, and affective symptoms of schizophrenia.

Nigrostriatal dopamine pathway

Another key dopamine pathway in the brain is the **nigrostriatal dopamine pathway**, which projects from dopaminergic cell bodies in the brainstem substantia nigra via axons terminating in the basal ganglia or striatum (Figure 1-30). The nigrostriatal dopamine pathway is a part of the extrapyramidal nervous system, and controls motor movements. Deficiencies in dopamine in this pathway cause movement disorders, including Parkinson's disease, characterized by rigidity, akinesia/bradykinesia (i.e., lack of movement or slowing of movement), and tremor. Dopamine deficiency in the basal ganglia can also produce akathisia (a type of restlessness) and dystonia (twisting movements, especially of the face and neck). These movement disorders can be replicated by drugs that block dopamine-2 receptors in this pathway and will be discussed briefly in Chapter 2.

Hyperactivity of dopamine in the nigrostriatal pathway is thought to underlie various hyperkinetic movement disorders such as chorea, dyskinesias, and tics. Chronic blockade of dopamine-2 receptors in this pathway may result in a hyperkinetic movement disorder known as neuroleptic-induced tardive dyskinesia. This will also be discussed briefly in Chapter 2. In schizophrenia, the nigrostriatal pathway in untreated patients may be relatively preserved (Figure 1-30).

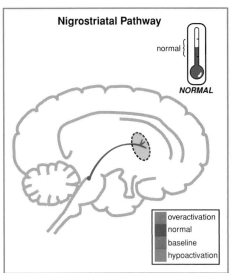

FIGURE 1-30 Nigrostriatal dopamine pathway. The nigrostriatal dopamine pathway projects from the substantia nigra to the basal ganglia or striatum. It is part of the extrapyramidal nervous system and plays a key role in regulating movements. When dopamine is deficient, it can cause parkinsonism with tremor, rigidity, and akinesia/bradykinesia. When DA is in excess, it can cause hyperkinetic movements like tics and dyskinesias. In untreated schizophrenia, activation of this pathway is believed to be "normal."

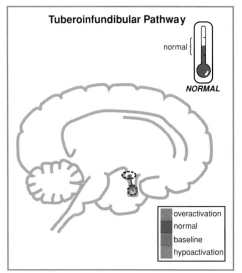

FIGURE 1-31 Tuberoinfundibular dopamine pathway. The tuberoinfundibular dopamine pathway from hypothalamus to anterior pituitary regulates prolactin secretion into the circulation. Dopamine inhibits prolactin secretion. In untreated schizophrenia, activation of this pathway is believed to be "normal."

Tuberoinfundibular dopamine pathway

The dopamine neurons that project from the hypothalamus to the anterior pituitary are known as the tuberoinfundibular dopamine pathway (Figure 1-31). Normally, these neurons are active and **inhibit** prolactin release. In the postpartum state, however, the activity of these dopamine neurons is decreased. Prolactin levels can therefore rise during breast-feeding so that lactation will occur. If the functioning of tuberoinfundibular dopamine neurons is disrupted by lesions or drugs, prolactin levels can also rise. Elevated prolactin levels are associated with galactorrhea (breast secretions), amenorrhea (loss of ovulation and menstrual periods), and possibly other problems such as sexual dysfunction. Such problems can occur after treatment with many antipsychotic drugs that block dopamine-2 receptors and will be discussed further in Chapter 2. In untreated schizophrenia, the function of the tuberoinfundibular pathway may be relatively preserved (Figure 1-31).

Thalamic dopamine pathway

A dopamine pathway that innervates the thalamus in primates has recently been described. It arises from multiple sites, including the periaqueductal gray matter, ventral mesencephalon, various hypothalamic nuclei, and lateral parabrachial nucleus (Figure 1-24). Its function is still under investigation but may be involved in sleep and arousal mechanisms by gating information passing through the thalamus to the cortex and other brain areas. There is no evidence at this point for abnormal functioning of this dopamine pathway in schizophrenia.

The integrated dopamine hypothesis of schizophrenia

Putting all this information together, the integrated dopamine hypothesis of schizophrenia attempts to explain all of the major symptoms of this disorder by dysregulation of either the mesolimbic dopamine pathway or the mesocortical dopamine pathway, with relative preservation of functioning of the nigrostriatal, tuberoinfundibular, and thalamic dopamine pathways (Figure 1-32). Specifically, positive symptoms of psychosis are hypothesized to be due to hyperactive mesolimbic dopamine neurons and negative, cognitive, and affective symptoms of schizophrenia are hypothesized to be due to underactivity of mesocortical dopamine neurons and their projections to prefrontal cortex (Figure 1-32). Underactive mesolimbic dopamine neurons may also contribute to reward-related negative symptoms in schizophrenia.

Glutamate

In recent years, the neurotransmitter glutamate has attained a key theoretical role in the pathophysiology of schizophrenia. It is also now a key target of novel psychopharmacological agents for future treatments of schizophrenia. In order to understand theories about glutamate in schizophrenia, how the malfunctioning of glutamate systems impacts dopamine systems in schizophrenia, and how glutamate systems might become important targets of new therapeutic drugs for schizophrenia, it is necessary to review the regulation of glutamate neurotransmission. Glutamate is the major excitatory neurotransmitter in the central nervous system and sometimes considered to be the "master switch" of the brain, since it can excite and turn on virtually all CNS neurons. The synthesis, metabolism, receptor regulation and key pathways of glutamate are therefore critical to the functioning of the brain and will be reviewed here.

Glutamate synthesis

Glutamate or glutamic acid is a neurotransmitter that is an amino acid. Its predominant use is not as a neurotransmitter but as an amino acid building block for protein biosynthesis. When used as a neurotransmitter, it is synthesized from glutamine in glial cells, which also assist in the recycling and regeneration of more glutamate following glutamate release during neurotransmission. Thus, glutamate is first released from synaptic vesicles that store this neurotransmitter in glutamate neurons and secondly taken up into neighboring glial cells by a reuptake pump known as an excitatory amino acid transporter (EAAT) (Figure 1-33A). The presynaptic glutamate neuron and the postsynaptic site of glutamate neurotransmission may also have EAATs (not shown in the figures), but these EAATs do not appear to play as important a role in glutamate recycling and regeneration as the EAATs in glial cells (Figure 1-33A).

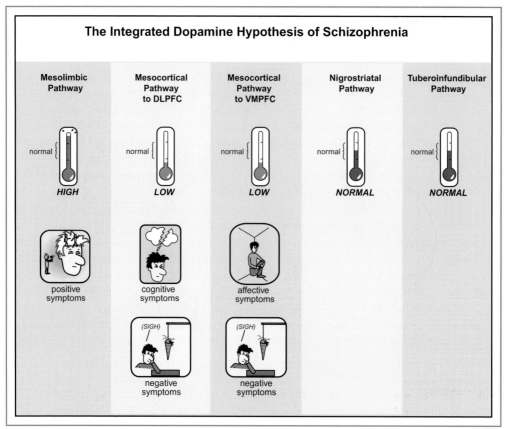

The Integrated Dopamine Hypothesis of Schizophrenia

FIGURE 1-32 Integrated dopamine hypothesis of schizophrenia. The majority of symptoms associated with schizophrenia may be explained by dysregulation of dopaminergic pathways; specifically by hyperactivity of the mesolimbic dopamine pathway (positive symptoms), hypoactivity of the mesocortical dopamine pathway to dorsolateral prefrontal cortex (DLPFC) (cognitive and negative symptoms), and hypoactivity of the mesocortical dopamine pathway to ventromedial prefrontal cortex (VMPFC) (affective and negative symptoms). The nigrostriatal and tuberoinfundibular dopamine pathways, though affected by antipsychotics used to treat schizophrenia, are believed to be "normal" in untreated schizophrenia.

Next, glutamate is converted into glutamine inside of glial cells by an enzyme known as glutamine synthetase (arrow 3 in Figure 1-33B). Glutamine is released from glial cells via reverse transport by a pump or transporter known as a specific neutral amino acid transporter (glial SNAT and arrow 4 in Figure 1-33C). Glutamine may also be transported out of glial cells by a second transporter known as a glial alanine-serine-cysteine transporter or ASC-T (not shown). When glial SNATs and ASC-Ts operate in the inward direction, they transport glutamine and other amino acids into the glial cell. Here, they are reversed, so that glutamine can get out of the glial cell and hop a ride into a neuron via a different type of neuronal SNAT operating inwardly in a reuptake manner (arrow 5 in Figure 1-33C).

Once inside the neuron, glutamine is converted into glutamate by an enzyme in mitochondria called glutaminase (arrow 6 in Figure 1-33D). Glutamate is then transported into synaptic vesicles via a vesicular glutamate transporter (vGluT, arrow 7 in Figure 1-33D),

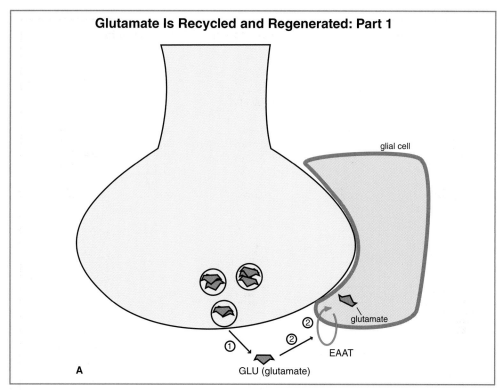

FIGURE 1-33A Glutamate is recycled and regenerated, part 1. After release of glutamate from the presynaptic neuron (1), it is taken up into glial cells via the EAAT, or excitatory amino acid transporter (2).

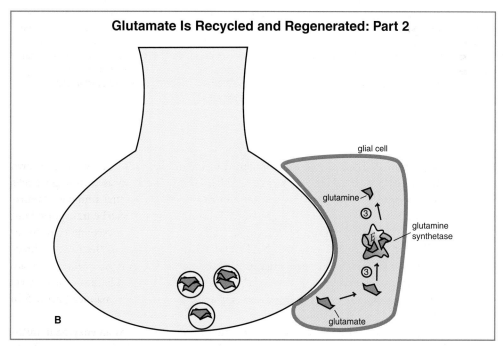

FIGURE 1-33B Glutamate is recycled and regenerated, part 2. Once inside the glial cell, glutamate is converted into glutamine by the enzyme glutamine synthetase (3).

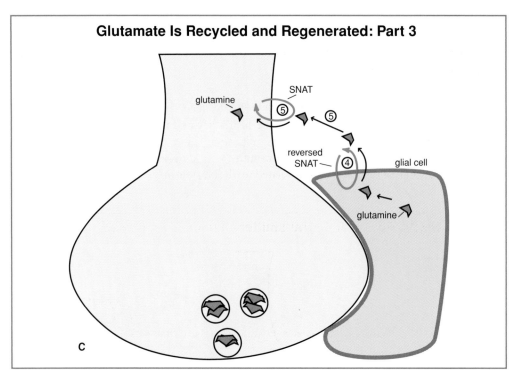

FIGURE 1-33C Glutamate is recycled and regenerated, part 3. Glutamine is released from glial cells by a specific neutral amino acid transporter (glial SNAT) through the process of reverse transport (4), and then taken up by SNATs on glutamate neurons (5).

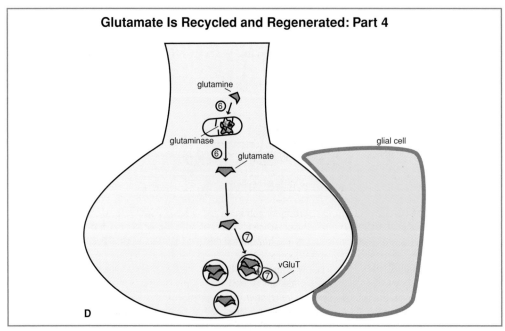

FIGURE 1-33D Glutamate is recycled and regenerated, part 4. Glutamine is converted into glutamate within the presynaptic glutamate neuron by the enzyme glutaminase (6) and taken up into synaptic vesicles by the vesicular glutamate transporter (vGluT), where it is stored for future release.

where it is stored for subsequent release during neurotransmission. Once released, glutamate's actions are stopped not by enzymatic breakdown, like in other neurotransmitter systems, but by removal by EAATs on neurons or glia, and the whole cycle is started again (Figure 1-33A through D).

Synthesis of glutamate cotransmitters glycine and d-serine

Glutamate systems are curious in that one of the key receptors for glutamate requires a cotransmitter in addition to glutamate in order to function. That receptor is the NMDA receptor, described below, and the cotransmitter is either the amino acid glycine (Figure 1-34), or another amino acid closely related to glycine, known as d-serine (Figure 1-35).

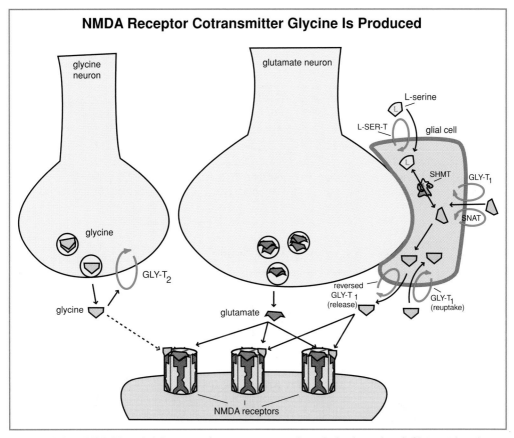

FIGURE 1-34 NMDA (N-methyl-d-aspartate) receptor cotransmitter glycine is produced. Glutamate's actions at NMDA receptors are dependent in part upon the presence of a cotransmitter, either glycine or d-serine. Glycine can be derived directly from dietary amino acids and transported into glial cells either by a glycine transporter (GlyT1) or by a specific neutral amino acid transporter (SNAT). Glycine can also be produced both in glycine neurons and in glial cells. Glycine neurons provide only a small amount of the glycine at glutamate synapses, because most of the glycine released by glycine neurons is used only at glycine synapses and then taken back up into presynaptic glycine neuron via the glycine 2 transporter (GLY-T2) before much glycine can diffuse to glutamate synapses. Glycine produced by glial cells plays a larger role at glutamate synapses. Glycine is produced in glial cells when the amino acid l-serine is taken up into glial cells via the l-serine transporter (l-SER-T), and then converted into glycine by the enzyme serine hydroxy methyl transferase (SHMT). Glycine from glial cells is released into the glutamate synapse through reverse transport by the glycine 1 transporter (GLY-T1). Extracellular glycine is then transported back into glial cells via a reuptake pump, namely GLY-T1.

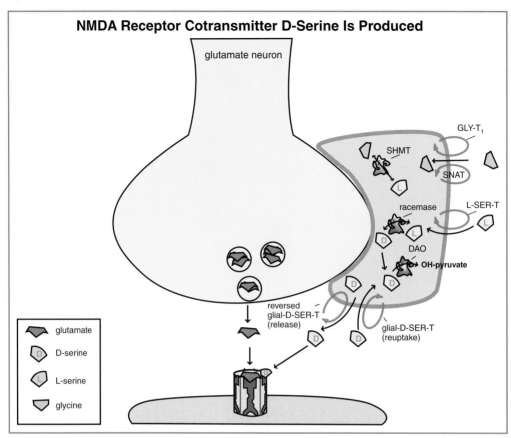

NMDA Receptor Cotransmitter D-Serine Is Produced

FIGURE 1-35 NMDA receptor cotransmitter d-serine is produced. Glutamate requires the presence of either glycine or d-serine at N-methyl-d-aspartate (NMDA) receptors in order to exert some of its effects there. In glial cells, the enzyme serine racemase converts l-serine into d-serine, which is then released into the glutamate synapse via reverse transport on the glial d-serine transporter (glial d-SER-T). l-serine's presence in glial cells is a result either of its transport there via the l-serine transporter (l-SER-T) or its conversion into l-serine from glycine via the enzyme serine hydroxy methyl transferase (SHMT). Once d-serine is released into the synapse, it is taken back up into the glial cell by a reuptake pump, namely d-SER-T. Excess d-serine within the glial cell can be destroyed by the enzyme d-amino acid oxidase (DAO), which converts d-serine into hydroxy-pyruvate (OH-pyruvate).

Glycine is not known to be synthesized by glutamate neurons, so glutamate neurons must get the glycine they need for their NMDA receptors either from glycine neurons or from glial cells (Figure 1-34). Glycine neurons release glycine, but they contribute only a small amount of glycine to glutamate synapses, since glycine is unable to diffuse very far from neighboring glycine neurons because the glycine they release is taken back up into those neurons by a type of glycine reuptake pump known as the type 2 glycine transporter, or Gly-T2 (Figure 1-34).

Thus, neighboring glial cells are thought to be the source of most of the glycine available for glutamate synapses. Glycine itself can be taken up into glial cells from the extracellular space or bloodstream by a type 1 glycine transporter, or Gly-T1 (Figure 1-34). Glycine can also be taken up into glial cells by a glial SNAT. Glycine is not known to be stored within synaptic vesicles of glial cells, but as we will learn below, the companion neurotransmitter d-serine is thought to be stored within some type of synaptic vesicle in glial cells. Glycine in the cytoplasm of glial cells is nevertheless somehow available for release into synapses, and it escapes from glial cells by riding outside them and into the glutamate synapse on a reversed Gly-T1 transporter (Figure 1-34). Once outside, glycine can get right back into the glial cell by an inwardly directed Gly-T1, which functions as a reuptake pump and is the main mechanism responsible for terminating the action of synaptic glycine (Figure 1-34). Later, in Chapter 2, we will discuss novel treatments for schizophrenia that boost glycine action and thus glutamate action at NMDA receptors; these are in testing and include inhibitors of the key glycine transporter Gly-T1.

Glycine can also be synthesized from the amino acid l-serine, derived from the extracellular space, bloodstream, and diet; transported into the glial cell by an l-serine transporter (SER-T); and converted from l-serine into glycine by the glial enzyme serine hydroxy methyl transferase (SHMT) (Figure 1-34). This enzyme works in both directions, either converting l-serine into glycine or glycine into l-serine.

How is the cotransmitter d-serine produced? D-serine is unusual in that it is a d-amino acid, whereas the twenty known essential amino acids are all l-amino acids, including d-serine's mirror image amino acid l-serine. It just so happens that d-serine has high affinity for the glycine site on NMDA receptors and that glial cells are equipped with an enzyme that can convert regular l-serine into the neurotransmitting amino acid d-serine by means of an enzyme that can go back and forth between d and l serine known as d-serine racemase (Figure 1-35). Thus, d-serine can be derived either from glycine or from l-serine, both of which can be transported into glial cells by their own transporters. Glycine is converted to l-serine by the enzyme SHMT and l-serine is converted into d-serine by the enzyme d-serine racemase (Figure 1-35). Interestingly, the d-serine so produced may be stored in some sort of vesicle in the glial cell for subsequent release on a reversed glial d-serine transporter (or d-SER-T) for neurotransmitting purposes at glutamate synapses containing NMDA receptors. D-serine's actions are terminated not only by synaptic reuptake via the inwardly acting glial d-SER-T but also by the enzyme d-amino acid oxidase (DAO), which converts d-serine into hydroxypyruvate (Figure 1-35). Below, an activator of DAO made by the brain, known not surprisingly as d-amino acid oxidase activator (DAOA), is discussed. The gene that makes DAOA may be one of the important regulatory genes that contribute to the genetic basis of schizophrenia, as explained below in the section on the neurodevelopmental hypothesis of schizophrenia.

Glutamate receptors

There are several types of glutamate receptors (Figure 1-36 and Table 1-11), including the neuronal presynaptic reuptake pump (excitatory amino acid transporter, or EAAT) and the vesicular transporter for glutamate into synaptic vesicles (vGluT). Shown also on the presynaptic neuron as well as the postsynaptic neuron are metabotropic glutamate receptors (Figure 1-36). Metabotropic glutamate receptors are linked to G proteins.

There are at least eight subtypes of metabotropic glutamate receptors, which are organized into three separate groups (Table 1-11). Research suggests that the metabotropic receptors of groups II and III can occur presynaptically, where they function as autoreceptors to block glutamate release (Figure 1-37). Drugs that stimulate these presynaptic autoreceptors as agonists may therefore reduce glutamate release and be potentially useful as anticonvulsants and mood stabilizers and also in protecting against glutamate excitotoxicity, as explained below. Group I metabotropic glutamate receptors may be located

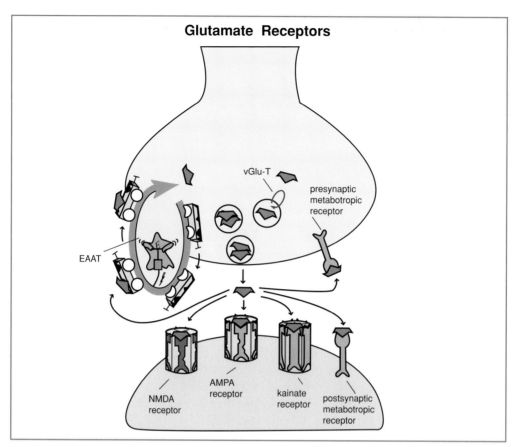

Glutamate Receptors

FIGURE 1-36 Glutamate receptors. Shown here are receptors for glutamate that regulate its neurotransmission. The excitatory amino acid transporter (EAAT) exists presynaptically and is responsible for clearing excess glutamate out of the synapse. The vesicular transporter for glutamate (v-Glu-T) transports glutamate into synaptic vesicles, where it is stored until used in a future neurotransmission. Metabotropic glutamate receptors (linked to G-proteins) can occur either pre- or postsynaptically. Three types of postsynaptic glutamate receptors are linked to ion channels, and are known as ligand-gated ion channels: N-methyl-d-aspartate (NMDA) receptors, alpha-amino-3-hydroxy-5-methyl-4-isoxazolepropionic acid (AMPA) receptors, and kainate receptors, all named for the agonists that bind to them.

predominantly postsynaptically, where they hypothetically interact with other postsynaptic glutamate receptors to facilitate and strengthen responses mediated by ligand-gated ion channel receptors for glutamate during excitatory glutamatergic neurotransmission (Figure 1-36).

NMDA, AMPA (alpha-amino-3-hydroxy-5-methyl-4-isoxazole-propionic acid), and kainate receptors for glutamate, named after the agonists that selectively bind to them, are all members of the ligand-gated ion channel family of receptors (Figure 1-36 and Table 1-11). These ligand-gated ion channels are also known as ionotropic receptors or ion channel–linked receptors. They all tend to be postsynaptic and work together to modulate excitatory postsynaptic neurotransmission triggered by glutamate. Specifically, AMPA and kainate receptors may mediate fast, excitatory neurotransmission, allowing sodium to enter the neuron to depolarize it. NMDA receptors in the resting state are normally blocked by

TABLE 1-11 Types of glutamate receptors

Metabotropic

Group I mGluR1
          mGluR5

Group II mGluR2
           mGluR3

Group III mGluR4
            mGluR6
            mGluR7
            mGluR8

Ionotropic (ligand-gated ion channels; ion channel–linked receptors)

Functional class	gene family	agonists	antagonists
AMPA	GluR1	glutamate	
	GluR2	AMPA	
	GluR3	kainate	
	GluR4		
Kainate	GluR5	glutamate	
	GluR6	kainate	
	GluR7		
	KA1		
	KA2		
NMDA	NR1	glutamate	
	NR2A	aspartate	
	NR2B	NMDA	MK801
	NR2C		ketamine
	NR2D		PCP (phencyclidine)

magnesium, which plugs its calcium channel. NMDA receptors are an interesting type of "coincidence detector" that can open to let calcium into the neuron to trigger postsynaptic actions from glutamate neurotransmission only when three things occur at the same time: glutamate occupies its binding site on the NMDA receptor, glycine or d-serine binds to its site on the NMDA receptor, and depolarization occurs, allowing the magnesium plug to be removed. Some of the many important signals by NMDA receptors that are activated when NMDA calcium channels are opened include not only long-term potentiation and synaptic plasticity but also excitotoxicity, as explained later in this chapter.

Key glutamate pathways in the brain and the NMDA receptor hypofunction hypothesis of schizophrenia

Glutamate is an ubiquitous excitatory neurotransmitter that seems to be able to excite nearly any neuron in the brain; that is why it is sometimes called the "master switch." Nevertheless, there are several specific glutamatergic pathways that are of particular relevance to psychopharmacology and especially to the pathophysiology of schizophrenia (Figure 1-38). These five pathways all relate to glutamatergic pyramidal neurons in the prefrontal cortex.

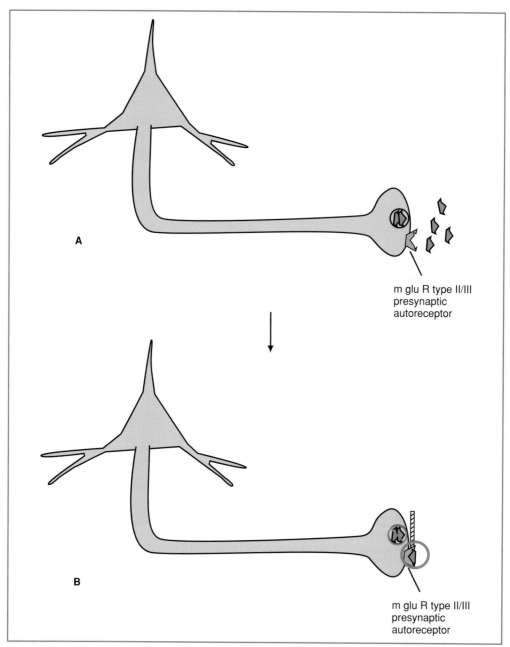

FIGURE 1-37A and B Metabotropic glutamate autoreceptors. Groups II and III metabotropic glutamate receptors can exist presynaptically as autoreceptors to regulate the release of glutamate. When glutamate builds up in the synapse (**A**), it is available to bind to the autoreceptor, which then inhibits glutamate release (**B**).

Corticobrainstem glutamate pathways and the NMDA receptor hypofunction hypothesis of schizophrenia

A very important descending glutamatergic pathway projects from cortical pyramidal neurons mostly in lamina 5 to brainstem neurotransmitter centers, including the raphe for serotonin, the ventral tegmental area (VTA) and substantia nigra for dopamine, and the

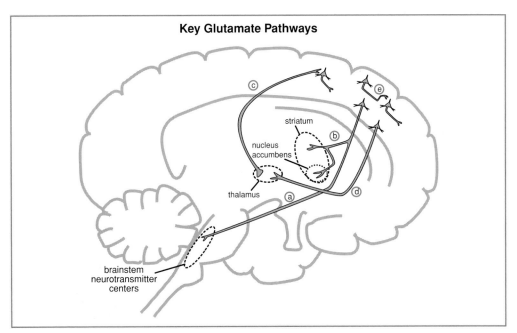

Key Glutamate Pathways

FIGURE 1-38 Five glutamate pathways in the brain. Although glutamate can have actions at virtually all neurons in the brain, there are five glutamate pathways particularly relevant to schizophrenia. (a) The **cortical brainstem glutamate projection** is a descending pathway that projects from cortical pyramidal neurons in the prefrontal cortex to brainstorm neurotransmitter centers (raphe, locus coeruleus, ventral tegmental area, substantia nigra) and regulates neurotransmitter release. (b) Another descending glutamatergic pathway projects from the prefrontal cortex to the striatum (**corticostriatal glutamate pathway**) and to the nucleus accumbens (corticoaccumbens glutamate pathway), and constitutes the "corticostriatal" portion of cortico-striatal-thalamic loops. (c) **Thalamocortical glutamate pathways** are pathways that ascend from the thalamus and innervate pyramidal neurons in the cortex. (d) **Corticothalamic glutamate pathways** descend from the prefrontal cortex to the thalamus. (e) Intracortical pyramidal neurons can communicate with each other via the neurotransmitter glutamate. These pathways are known as **corticocortical glutamatergic pathways**.

locus coeruleus for norepinephrine (pathway a in Figure 1-38). This pathway is the cortical brainstem glutamate projection and is a key regulator of neurotransmitter release. Specifically, this descending corticobrainstem glutamate pathway normally acts as a brake on the mesolimbic dopamine pathway. It does this by communicating with these dopamine neurons through an inhibitory GABA interneuron in the VTA (Figure 1-39A). This normally results in tonic inhibition of dopamine release from the mesolimbic pathway (Figure 1-39A).

A major current hypothesis for schizophrenia involves NMDA receptors in this pathway. The NMDA receptor hypofunction hypothesis of schizophrenia arises from observations that when NMDA receptors are made hypofunctional by means of the NMDA receptor antagonist phencyclidine (PCP), this produces a psychotic condition in normal humans very similar to the positive symptoms of schizophrenia, including hallucinations and delusions. To a lesser extent, the NMDA receptor antagonist ketamine can also produce a schizophrenia-like psychosis in normals.

Such observations have led to the hypothesis that NMDA receptors specifically in the corticobrainstem glutamate projection might be hypoactive in untreated schizophrenia and thus cannot do their job of tonically inhibiting mesolimbic dopamine neurons. When this happens, mesolimbic dopamine hyperactivity is the result. This is theoretically

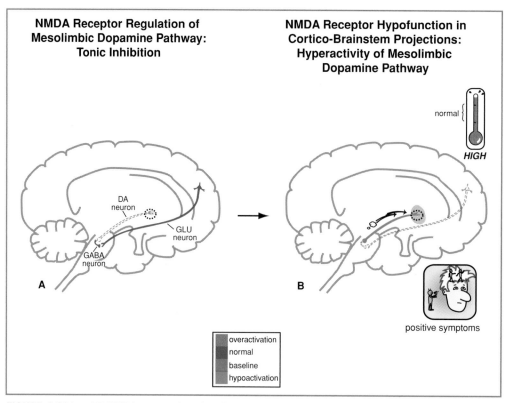

FIGURE 1-39A and B NMDA receptor hypofunction hypothesis and positive symptoms of schizophrenia.
(A) The cortical brainstem glutamate projection communicates with the mesolimbic dopamine pathway via a gamma aminobutyric acid (GABA) interneuron in the ventral tegmental area. Excitatory glutamate stimulates N-methyl-d-aspartate (NMDA) receptors on the interneuron, causing GABA release, and GABA, in turn, inhibits release of dopamine from the mesolimbic dopamine pathway; thus the descending glutamatergic pathway normally acts as a brake on the mesolimbic dopamine pathway. (B) If NMDA receptors in the cortical brainstem glutamate projection are *hypo*active, then the downstream effect of tonic inhibition of the mesolimbic dopamine pathway will not occur, leading to *hyper*activity in this pathway. This is the theoretical biological basis for the mesolimbic dopamine hyperactivity thought to be associated with the positive symptoms of psychosis.

the consequence of corticobrainstem glutamate hypoactivity at NMDA receptors (Figure 1-39B).

Thus the mesolimbic dopamine hypothesis of positive symptoms of schizophrenia shown in Figures 1-25B and 1-26 may be explained by the NMDA receptor hypofunction hypothesis of schizophrenia shown in Figure 1-39B. That is, mesolimbic dopamine hyperactivity that produces positive symptoms of schizophrenia may actually be the consequence of NMDA receptor hypoactivation in corticobrainstem glutamate projections, as shown in Figure 1-39B.

What is so attractive about the NMDA receptor hypofunction hypothesis of schizophrenia is that unlike amphetamine which activates only positive symptoms, PCP also mimics the cognitive, negative and affective symptoms of schizophrenia. That is, normal humans who take PCP and render their NMDA receptors hypofunctional not only experience positive symptoms such as delusions and hallucinations, but also affective symptoms such as blunted affect, negative symptoms such as social withdrawal, and cognitive

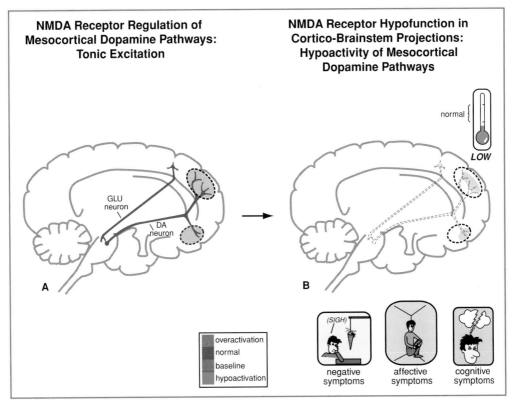

NMDA Receptor Regulation of Mesocortical Dopamine Pathways: Tonic Excitation

NMDA Receptor Hypofunction in Cortico-Brainstem Projections: Hypoactivity of Mesocortical Dopamine Pathways

GLU neuron

DA neuron

normal

LOW

overactivation
normal
baseline
hypoactivation

(SIGH)

negative symptoms

affective symptoms

cognitive symptoms

A

B

FIGURE 1-40A and B NMDA receptor hypofunction hypothesis and negative, cognitive, and affective symptoms of schizophrenia. (**A**) The cortical brainstem glutamate projection communicates directly with the mesocortical dopamine pathway in the ventral tegmental area, normally causing tonic excitation. (**B**) If N-methyl-d-aspartate (NMDA) receptors in cortical brainstem glutamate projections are hypoactive, tonic excitation here is lost and mesocortical dopamine pathways become hypoactive, potentially explaining the cognitive, negative, and affective symptoms of schizophrenia.

symptoms such as executive dysfunction. These additional clinical observations have led to the idea that NMDA receptors in corticobrainstem glutamate projections that regulate mesocortical dopamine pathways may also be hypoactive in schizophrenia.

How can this be explained? Normally, these descending corticobrainstem glutamate neurons act as accelerators to mesocortical dopamine neurons. Unlike the actions of corticobrainstem glutamate neurons on mesolimbic dopamine neurons shown in Figure 1-39A, where they act via an intermediary GABA interneuron, corticobrainstem glutamate neurons synapse directly on those dopamine neurons in the ventral tegmental area that project to the cortex, those so-called mesocortical dopamine neurons (Figure 1-40A). This means that corticobrainstem glutamate neurons normally function as accelerators of these mesocortical dopamine neurons; therefore they excite them tonically (Figure 1-40A).

The consequence of this neuronal circuitry is that when corticobrainstem projections to mesocortical dopamine neurons have NMDA receptor hypoactivity, they lose their excitatory drive and become hypoactive, as shown in Figure 1-40B. This could hypothetically explain why mesocortical dopamine neurons are hypoactive and thus their link to the cognitive, negative, and affective symptoms of schizophrenia, as shown in Figures 1-27B, 1-28B, and 1-29.

Corticostriatal glutamate pathways

A second descending glutamatergic output from pyramidal neurons projecting to the striatum is shown as pathway b in Figure 1-38. This pathway is known as the corticostriatal glutamate pathway when it projects to the striatum itself or the corticoaccumbens glutamate pathway when it projects to a specific area of the ventral striatum known as the nucleus accumbens. In either case, it originates from pyramidal neurons in lamina 5 of the cortex. This corticostriatal pathway is the first leg of cortico-striatal-thalamic-cortical (CSTC) loops, which are the brain's engines for behavioral and functional outputs.

Normally, this corticostriatal glutamate projection to the striatum terminates on GABA neurons in the striatum (number 1 in Figure 1-41A), which in turn project to the thalamus (number 2 in Figure 1-41A). In the thalamus, these GABA neurons create a "sensory filter" to prevent too much of the sensory traffic coming into the thalamus from escaping to the cortex, where it may confuse or overwhelm cortical information processing (arrow 3 in Figure 1-41A).

Dopamine functions in this CSTC loop to inhibit the GABA neurons projecting to the thalamus, thus reducing the effectiveness of the thalamic filter (Figure 1-41B). This opposes the excitatory input of glutamate from corticostriatal glutamate projections to the striatum (Figures 1-41A and B).

Thalamocortical glutamate pathways

An ascending glutamate pathway starts from the thalamus and innervates pyramidal neurons and is known as the thalamocortical pathway (pathway c in Figure 1-38). This is the return leg of the CSTC loop, namely from thalamus to cortex, and provides not only feedback to the original pyramidal cell "cortical engine" from information processing that occurs in the CSTC loop (see number 3 in Figure 1-41A), but also input diffusely throughout the cortex to numerous other pyramidal neurons and their CSTC loops (see arrow 3 in Figure 1-41C). A properly functioning thalamic filter prevents too much sensory input from penetrating the thalamus into the cortex, so that information processing can occur in an orderly manner (Figure 1-41C).

How does NMDA receptor hypofunction affect information processing in CSTC loops? First, when descending corticobrainstem glutamate pathways have hypofunctioning NMDA receptors in the ventral tegmental area, this creates mesolimbic dopamine hyperactivity and positive symptoms of psychosis, as already explained above and illustrated in Figure 1-39B. The effects of this on CSTC loops are shown in Figure 1-41D, where dopamine hyperactivity reduces the thalamic filter and permits the escape of excessive sensory information coming into the thalamus, thus allowing it to get into the cortex by means of ascending thalamocortical neurons.

If this were not bad enough, there is hypothetical NMDA receptor hypofunction in the descending corticostriatal glutamate pathway as well (Figure 1-41E). This reduces the excitatory drive on the GABA neurons that create the thalamic filter. Coupled with the excessive dopamine drive from mesolimbic neurons, the thalamic filter fails, and too much information escapes diffusely into the cortex, where it can cause cortical manifestations of hallucinations or may also create other cortical symptoms such as cognitive, affective, and negative symptoms of schizophrenia (Figure 1-41E).

Corticothalamic glutamate pathways

A third descending glutamatergic pathway, mostly from lamina 6 in the cortex, projects directly to the thalamus, where it may provide sensory and other types of input

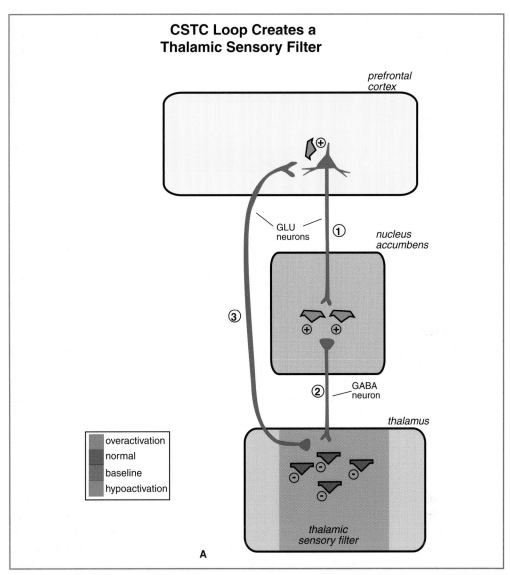

CSTC Loop Creates a Thalamic Sensory Filter

FIGURE 1-41A The cortico-striatal-thalamic-cortical loop creates a thalamic sensory filter. Pyramidal glutamatergic neurons descend from the prefrontal cortex to the striatum (1), where they terminate on gamma aminobutyric acid (GABA) neurons (2) that project to the thalamus. The release of GABA in the thalamus creates a sensory filter that prevents too much sensory information traveling through the thalamus from reaching the cortex, including the feedback thalamocortical glutamate neurons that project back to the original cortical pyramidal neuron (3).

(pathway d in Figure 1-38). This is known as the corticothalamic pathway. This may represent some of the sensory input that arrives via glutamate neurons to the thalamus in Figure 1-41C, D, and E. Hypofunction of NMDA receptors at this level may also cause dysregulation of the information that arrives in the cortex due to sensory overload and a malfunctioning of cortical glutamate input directly to the thalamic filter (Figure 1-41E).

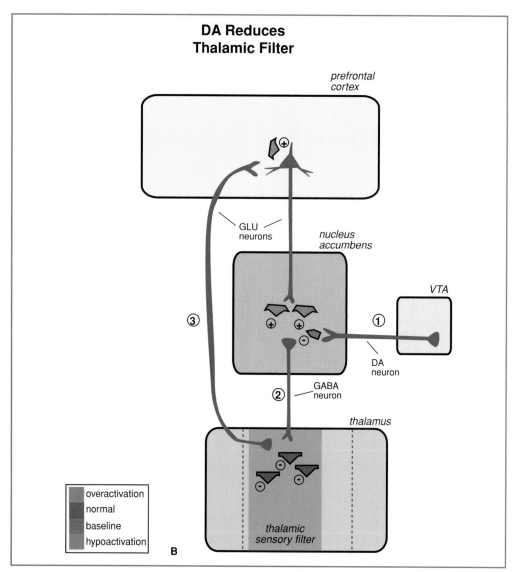

DA Reduces Thalamic Filter

FIGURE 1-41B Dopamine reduces the thalamic filter. Dopaminergic input to the nucleus accumbens via the mesolimbic dopamine pathway (1) has an inhibitory effect on gamma aminobutyric acid (GABA) neurons (2). Thus, dopamine input (1) reduces the stimulatory glutamatergic input to these neurons from the prefrontal cortex, and thereby reduces the effectiveness of the thalamic sensory filter since less GABA is released by GABA neurons projecting from the nucleus accumbens to the thalamus (2). This means that more sensory input can escape from the thalamus to the cortex (3).

Corticocortical glutamate pathways

One pyramidal neuron communicates with another via the neurotransmitter glutamate (Figure 1-38, pathway e). These pathways are known as corticocortical glutamatergic pathways.

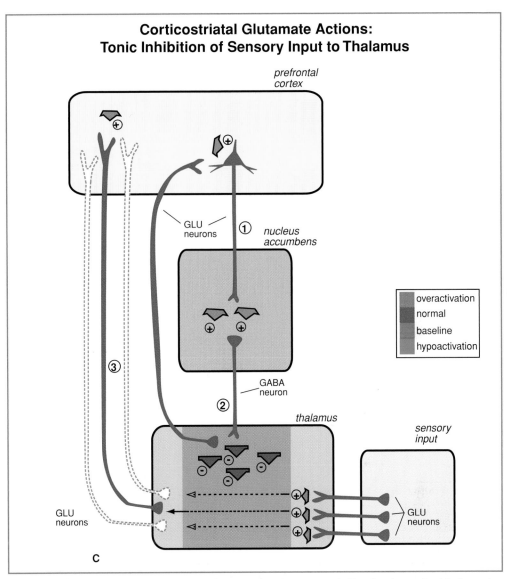

**Corticostriatal Glutamate Actions:
Tonic Inhibition of Sensory Input to Thalamus**

FIGURE 1-41C Tonic inhibition of sensory input from thalamus. A thalamic filter for sensory input to the cortex is set up by glutamate neurons projecting to nucleus accumbens (1), stimulating GABA release in the thalamus (2). When effective, this inhibitory GABA filters out most sensory input arriving in the thalamus, so that only selected types of sensory input are relayed to the cortex (3).

Cortical pyramidal neurons thus utilize glutamate to communicate back and forth: they not only send information to other pyramidal neurons with glutamate but also receive information from other neurons via glutamate (Figure 1-38). Glutamate is the main neurotransmitter utilized to send information as output from pyramidal neurons, but these neurons can receive a whole host of chemical neurotransmitting messages as input from other neurons.

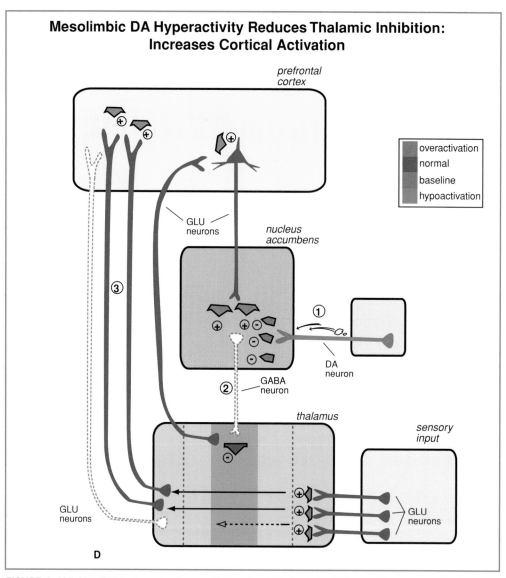

Mesolimbic DA Hyperactivity Reduces Thalamic Inhibition: Increases Cortical Activation

FIGURE 1-41D Mesolimbic dopamine hyperactivity reduces thalamic inhibition and increases cortical activation. The inhibitory effect of dopamine represented in Figure 1-41B is shown here as being much enhanced when this mesolimbic dopamine pathway is hyperactive (1). Too much dopamine activity in the nucleus accumbens (1), reduces GABA output to the thalamus (2), thus greatly reducing the effectiveness of the thalamic filter. When this occurs, more sensory input gets through the thalamic filter and increases the amount of cortical activation by ascending thalamocortical glutamate neurons (3). This definitely causes increased cortical activation and could potentially even cause overload in the prefrontal cortex, and positive symptoms of schizophrenia. See also Figure 1-41E.

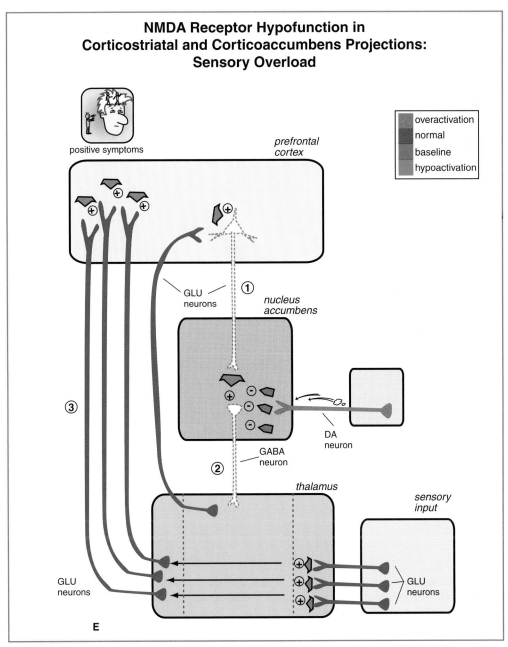

NMDA Receptor Hypofunction in Corticostriatal and Corticoaccumbens Projections: Sensory Overload

positive symptoms

prefrontal cortex

overactivation
normal
baseline
hypoactivation

GLU neurons

① nucleus accumbens

③

DA neuron

GABA neuron

②

thalamus

sensory input

GLU neurons

GLU neurons

E

FIGURE 1-41E N-methyl-d-aspartate (NMDA) receptor hypofunction in corticostriatal and corticoaccumbens projections: sensory overload. NMDA receptor hypofunction in glutamatergic corticostriatal and corticoaccumbens projections (1) reduces the excitatory drive on gamma aminobutyric acid (GABA) neurons that create the thalamic filter (2), which can lead to excess sensory information escaping to the cortex (3). When this NMDA receptor hypofunction (1) is coupled with hyperactivity of mesolimbic dopamine neurons (shown here on the right and also in Figure 1-41D), this can cause the thalamic filter (2) to fail to the point where so much sensory information reaches the cortex that positive symptoms of psychosis occur (3) (see positive symptom icon in the cortex).

In terms of the NMDA receptor hypofunction hypothesis of schizophrenia, it is not difficult to see how malfunctioning of glutamate input into cortical pyramidal neurons, not just from thalamocortical neurons (shown in Figure 1-41) but also from corticocortical neurons communicating within the cortex (shown in Figure 1-38) could contribute to symptoms of schizophrenia that theoretically reside in prefrontal cortex, such as cognitive, affective, and negative symptoms.

That is, normally corticocortical projections and loops between key areas of prefrontal cortex communicate effectively and process information efficiently (Figure 1-42A). When NMDA receptors are hypofunctional, this changes the nature of information processing such that corticocortical communication of one glutamatergic pyramidal cell to another becomes dysfunctional (Figure 1-42B). Theoretically, this can range from hypoactivation of the entire loop, as shown for the corticocortical loop between dorsolateral prefrontal cortex (DLPFC) and ventromedial prefrontal cortex (VMPFC) in Figure 1-42B, to over-activation of the entire loop as shown from VMPFC to orbitofrontal cortex (OFC) to partial overactivation with partial hypoactivation as shown for OFC to DLPFC in Figure 1-42B. Whatever the actual activation pattern, communication when NMDA receptors are hypofunctional can be faulty if not chaotic, thus, according to the NMDA receptor hypofunction hypothesis, leading to the symptoms of schizophrenia.

In summary, NMDA receptor hypofunction within the five major glutamate pathways described in Figure 1-38 can potentially explain not only the positive, negative, affective, and cognitive symptoms of schizophrenia but also how dopamine becomes dysregulated as a consequence of NMDA receptor hypofunction, and thus too active in the mesolimbic dopamine pathway for positive symptoms and too hypoactive in the mesocortical dopamine pathway for cognitive, affective, and negative symptoms of schizophrenia. Many contemporary theories on the genetic basis of schizophrenia now focus on the NMDA receptor, as discussed below, as do new drug development efforts for novel treatments of schizophrenia, discussed in Chapter 2.

Neurodegenerative hypothesis of schizophrenia

The presence of both functional and structural abnormalities demonstrated in neuroimaging studies of the brain of schizophrenics suggests that a neurodegenerative process with progressive loss of neuronal function may be ongoing during the course of schizophrenia (Figure 1-43). Numerous neurodegenerative processes are hypothesized, ranging from genetic programming of abnormal apoptosis and subsequent degeneration of critical neurons, to prenatal exposure to anoxia, toxins, infection, or malnutrition, to a process of neuronal loss known as excitotoxicity (Figure 1-43). If neurons are excited while mediating positive symptoms and then die off from a toxic process caused by excessive excitatory neurotransmission, this may lead to a residual burnout state and thus negative symptoms (Figure 1-43).

A neurodegenerative condition in schizophrenia is also suggested by the progressive nature of the course of this illness (Figure 1-44). Such a course is not consistent with simply being the result of a static and previously completed pathologic process. Thus, schizophrenia progresses from a largely asymptomatic stage prior to the teen years (phase I in Figure 1-44), to a prodromal stage of "oddness" and the onset of subtle negative symptoms in the late teens to early twenties (phase II in Figure 1-44). The active phase of the illness begins and continues throughout the twenties and thirties, with destructive positive symptoms characterized by an up-and-down course with treatment and relapse, never quite returning

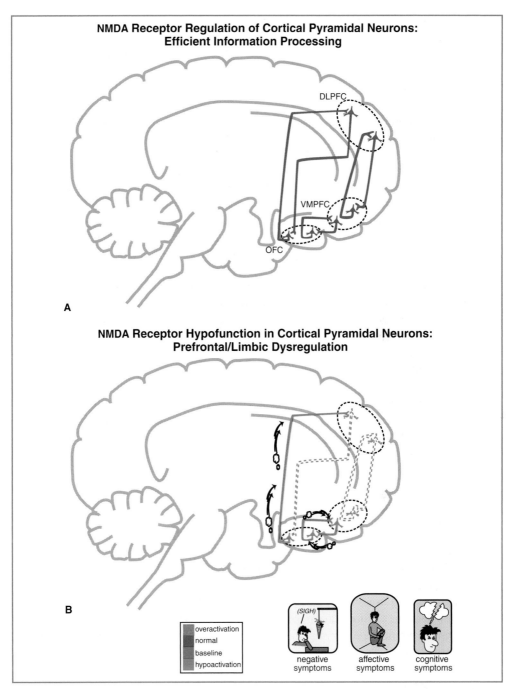

FIGURE 1-42A and B N-methyl-d-aspartate (NMDA) receptor regulation of corticocortical glutamate pathways.
(**A**) When NMDA receptors function normally, corticocortical glutamate loops communicate effectively and process information efficiently. (**B**) NMDA receptor hypofunction in cortical pyramidal neurons can impair communication between neurons by causing hypoactivation of loops [shown here, for example, between dorsolateral prefrontal cortex (DLPFC) and ventral medial prefrontal cortex (VMPFC)], hyperactivation of loops [shown here, for example, between orbitofrontal cortex (OFC) and VMPFC], and even partial hyperactivation with partial hypoactivation (shown here, for example, between OFC and DLPFC). Dysfunction of corticocortical glutamate pathways due to NMDA receptor hypofunction could be an underlying cause of schizophrenia symptoms.

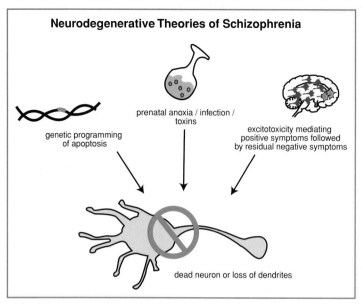

Neurodegenerative Theories of Schizophrenia

genetic programming
of apoptosis

prenatal anoxia / infection /
toxins

excitotoxicity mediating
positive symptoms followed
by residual negative symptoms

dead neuron or loss of dendrites

FIGURE 1-43 Neurodegenerative theories of schizophrenia. Neurodegenerative theories of schizophrenia posit that progressive loss of neuronal function – whether through loss of dendrites, destruction of synapses, or neuronal death – may underlie symptoms and progression of schizophrenia. Causes of neurodegeneration can range from predetermined genetic programming of neuronal or synaptic destruction; to fetal insults such as anoxia, infection, toxins, or maternal starvation; to glutamate-mediated excitotoxicity that initially can cause positive symptoms, and, as neurons die, lead to residual negative symptoms.

to the same level of functioning following acute relapses or exacerbations (phase III in Figure 1-44). Finally, the disease can go into a largely stable stage of poor social functioning and prominent negative and cognitive symptoms, with some ups and downs but at a considerable decline from baseline functioning, suggesting a more static phase of illness, sometimes called burnout, in the forties or later in life (phase IV in Figure 1-44).

The fact that a schizophrenic patient's responsiveness to antipsychotic treatment can change (and lessen) over the course of illness also suggests an ongoing neurodegenerative process of some kind. For example, the time it takes for a schizophrenic patient to go into remission increases with each successive psychotic relapse. Patients may be less responsive to antipsychotic treatment during successive episodes or exacerbations, such that residual symptoms remain as well as decrements in the patients' functional capacities. This development of treatment resistance during successive episodes of the illness suggests that "psychosis is hazardous to the brain." It thus seems possible that patients who receive early and effective continuous treatment may avoid disease progression or at least the development of treatment resistance.

One major idea that proposes to explain the downhill course of schizophrenia and the development of treatment resistance is that neurodegenerative events in schizophrenia may be mediated by a type of excessive action of the neurotransmitter glutamate that has come to be known as "excitotoxicity." The "excitotoxic hypothesis of schizophrenia" proposes that neurons degenerate because of excessive excitatory neurotransmission at glutamate neurons. This process of excitotoxicity is not only a hypothesis to explain neurodegeneration in schizophrenia; it has also been invoked as an explanation for neurodegeneration in any number of neurologic and psychiatric conditions, including Alzheimer's disease and other

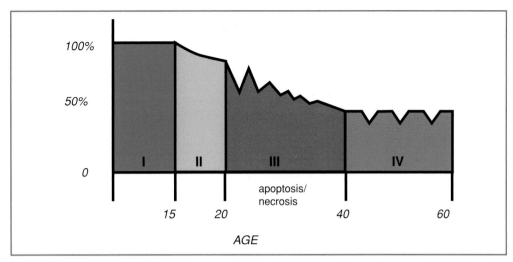

FIGURE 1-44 Stages of schizophrenia. The stages of schizophrenia are shown here over a lifetime. The progressive nature of schizophrenia, illustrated here, supports a neurodegenerative basis for the disorder. The patient has full functioning (100 percent) early in life, and is virtually asymptomatic (Stage I). However, during a prodromal phase (Stage II) starting in the teens, there may be odd behaviors and subtle negative symptoms. The acute phase of the illness usually announces itself fairly dramatically in the twenties (Stage III) with positive symptoms, remissions, and relapses but never quite getting back to previous levels of functioning. This is often a chaotic stage of illness with a progressive downhill course. The final phase of the illness may begin in the forties or later, with prominent negative and cognitive symptoms and some waxing and waning, but often more of a "burnout" stage of continuing disability. There may not necessarily be a continuing and relentless downhill course, but the patient may become progressively resistant to treatment with antipsychotic medications during this stage (Stage IV).

degenerative dementias, Parkinson's disease, amytrophic lateral sclerosis (ALS, or Lou Gehrig's disease), and even stroke.

Excitotoxicity and the glutamate system in neurodegenerative disorders such as schizophrenia

The NMDA subtype of glutamate receptor is thought to mediate both normal excitatory neurotransmission, leading to vital functions such as neuronal plasticity and long-term potentiation (Figure 1-45) as well as neurodegenerative excitotoxicity along the glutamate excitation spectrum shown in Figure 1-46. Excitotoxicity could be the final common pathway that leads to progressive worsening in any number of neurologic and psychiatric disorders characterized by a neurodegenerative course. The basic idea is that the normal process of excitatory neurotransmission runs amok, and instead of normal excitatory neurotransmission, things get out of hand and the neuron is literally excited to death (Figures 1-46 and 1-47). The excitotoxic mechanism is thought to begin with a pathologic process of overexcitation that may accompany symptoms such as psychosis, mania, or even panic (Figures 1-46 and 1-48). The storm of excitatory symptoms could be the trigger for reckless glutamate activity leading ultimately to neuronal death (Figure 1-47). The sequence of ever more dangerous excitatory neurotransmission could begin with potentially reversible excess calcium entering neurons during excitatory neurotransmission with glutamate, mediating positive symptoms of psychosis, and possibly allowing full recovery of the neuron (left-hand part of the spectrum in Figures 1-46 and 1-48). However, such a state of overexcitation could also lead to dangerous opening of the calcium channel, because if too much calcium

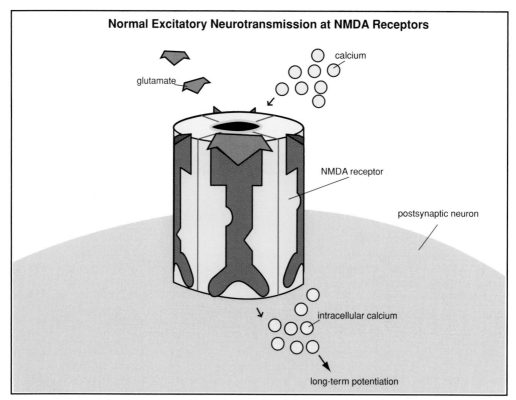

Normal Excitatory Neurotransmission at NMDA Receptors

calcium

glutamate

NMDA receptor

postsynaptic neuron

intracellular calcium

long-term potentiation

FIGURE 1-45 Normal excitatory neurotransmission at NMDA receptors. Shown here is normal excitatory neurotransmission at the N-methyl-d-aspartate (NMDA) type of glutamate receptor. The NMDA receptor is a ligand-gated ion channel. This fast transmitting ion channel is an excitatory calcium channel. Occupancy of NMDA glutamate receptors by glutamate causes calcium channels to open and the neuron to be excited for neurotransmission.

enters the cell through open channels, it would poison the cell due to calcium activation of intracellular enzymes (Figure 1-48) that form pesky free radicals (Figure 1-49). Initially, free radicals begin destroying just the dendrites that serve as postsynaptic targets of gluta-mate (Figure 1-50). However, too many free radicals would eventually overwhelm the cell with toxic actions on cellular membranes and organelles (Figure 1-51), ultimately killing the neuron.

A limited form of excitotoxicity may be useful as a "pruning" mechanism for normal maintenance of the dendritic tree, getting rid of cerebral "deadwood" like a good gardener; excitotoxicity to excess, however, is hypothesized to be a form of pruning out of control. This hypothetically results in various forms of neurodegeneration, ranging from slow, relentless neurodegenerative conditions such as schizophrenia and Alzheimer's disease to sudden, catastrophic neuronal death such as stroke (Figure 1-46).

Neurodevelopmental hypothesis and genetics of schizophrenia

Is schizophrenia acquired or inherited?

Many contemporary theories for the etiology of schizophrenia propose that this illness orig-inates from abnormalities in brain development. Some suggest that the problem is acquired

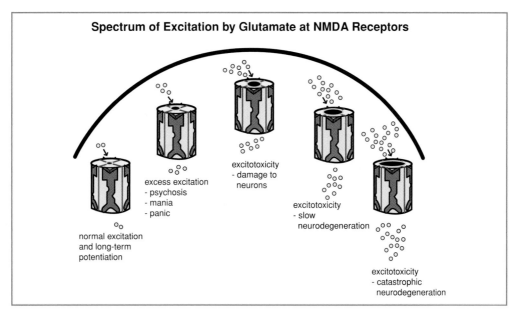

FIGURE 1-46 Spectrum of excitation by glutamate at N-methyl-d-aspartate (NMDA) receptors. A major hypothesis for the pathophysiology of neurologic and psychiatric disorders that run a neurodegenerative course is that glutamate may cause neuronal damage or death by a process of normal excitatory neurotransmission run amok, called excitotoxicity. The spectrum of excitation by glutamate ranges from normal neurotransmission, which is necessary for such neuronal activities as long-term potentiation, memory formation, and synaptogenesis; to an excessive amount of excitatory neurotransmission that may occur while a patient is experiencing pathologic symptoms such as psychosis, mania, or panic; to excitotoxicity that results in damage to dendrites but not neuronal death; to slow progressive excitotoxicity resulting in neuronal degeneration of many neurons over an extended period of time, as occurs in Alzheimer's disease or possibly schizophrenia; to sudden and catastrophic excitotoxicity causing neurodegeneration leading to loss of a large number of neurons at once, as in stroke.

from the fetal brain's environment, as shown in Figure 1-43. Schizophrenia may thus start with an acquired neurodegenerative process that interferes with neurodevelopment. For example, schizophrenia is increased in those with a fetal history of obstetric complications in the pregnant mother – ranging from viral infections to starvation to autoimmune processes and other such problems – suggesting that an insult to the brain early in fetal development could contribute to the cause of schizophrenia. These risk factors may all have the final common pathway of reducing nerve growth factors and also stimulating certain noxious processes that kill off critical neurons, such as cytokines, viral infection, hypoxia, trauma, starvation, or stress. This may be mediated by either apoptosis or necrosis.

Neuronal insult could also be mediated by excitotoxicity, as discussed earlier (Figures 1-46 through 1-51). In particular, if excitotoxicity occurred specifically in the ventral hippocampus before the completion of connections in the developing brain, some neurodevelopmental theories suggest that this could impact the development of the prefrontal cortex and result in dysconnectivity with the prefrontal cortex (Figure 1-52). Such an abnormal set of neuronal connections could be the biological substrate for symptoms in schizophrenia (Figure 1-52). The excitotoxicity that causes such dysconnectivity could be genetically programmed or environmentally triggered.

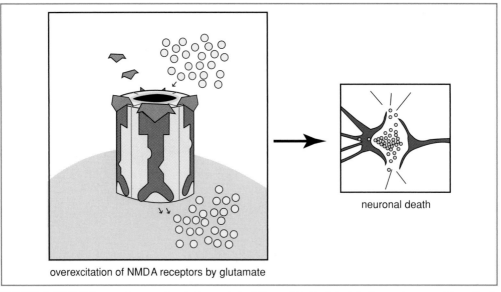

overexcitation of NMDA receptors by glutamate

neuronal death

FIGURE 1-47 Cellular events occurring during excitotoxicity, part 1. Excitotoxicity is a major current hypothesis for explaining a neuropathologic mechanism that could mediate the final common pathway of any number of neurologic and psychiatric disorders characterized by a neurodegenerative course. The basic idea is that the normal process of excitatory neurotransmission runs amok, and instead of normal excitatory neurotransmission, things get out of hand and the neuron is literally excited to death. The excitotoxic mechanism is thought to begin with a pathologic process that triggers excessive glutamate activity. This causes excessive opening of the calcium channel, shown here, beginning the process of poisoning of the cell by allowing too much calcium to enter it.

Genes that affect connectivity, synaptogenesis and NMDA receptors

Although abnormal neuronal connectivity can be triggered in many ways by the environment (Figure 1-43), it is increasingly believed that the neurodevelopmental processes underlying schizophrenia are mostly influenced by genes. Strong evidence for a genetic basis of schizophrenia comes from the classic schizophrenia twin studies showing that monozygotic twins are much more frequently concordant for schizophrenia than are dizygotic twins. For many years, scientists have therefore been trying to identify abnormal genes in schizophrenia. Once it was recognized that single genes do not directly cause schizophrenia or the behavioral symptoms of schizophrenia, attention turned to the discovery of "susceptibility" genes that code for subtle molecular abnormalities that could provide a genetic bias toward inefficient information processing in brain circuits mediating the symptoms of schizophrenia. A sufficient combination of such genetic bias, particularly when coupled with stressful input from the environment, is the modern formulation for how genes and the environment conspire to produce schizophrenia.

More than a dozen susceptibility genes have been identified, several of which have been reproducibly linked to schizophrenia (Table 1-12). The pathogenic mechanisms of the most prominent genes described by current genetic research in schizophrenia include abnormal neuronal connectivity, defective synaptogenesis, and dysregulation of the NMDA glutamate receptor (Figures 1-53 through 1-58). Four key genes that regulate neuronal connectivity and synaptogenesis in schizophrenia are shown in Figure 1-53. These are the genes for four key proteins: **BDNF** (brain-derived neurotrophic factor), a known trophic factor

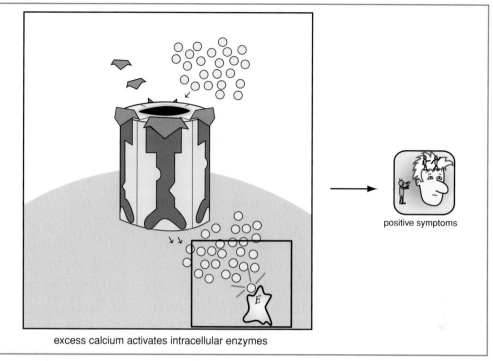

positive symptoms

excess calcium activates intracellular enzymes

FIGURE 1-48 Cellular events occurring during excitotoxicity, part 2. The internal milieu of a neuron is very sensitive to calcium, as a small increase in calcium concentration will alter the activities of various enzymes as well as cause alterations in neuronal membrane excitability. If calcium levels rise too much, then they will begin to activate enzymes that can be dangerous for the cell owing to their ability to trigger a destructive chemical cascade. The beginning of this process may be an underlying cause of pathologic symptoms of schizophrenia such as delusions and hallucinations.

dysbindin, also known as dystrobrevin-binding protein 1, involved in the formation of synaptic structures (Figures 1-53 and 1-55A and B); **neuregulin**, involved in neuronal migration (Figures 1-53 and 1-54B) and in the genesis of glial cells and subsequent myelination of neurons by these cells (Figure 1-54D); and **DISC-1** (disrupted in schizophrenia-1), aptly named for a disrupted gene linked to schizophrenia that makes a protein involved in neurogenesis (Figure 1-54A), neuronal migration (Figure 1-54B), and dendritic organization (Figures 1-53 and 1-54C).

It is not known exactly how these genes cause the hypothesized subtle molecular abnormalities that are thought to bias neuronal circuits towards schizophrenia or whether these genes make abnormal proteins or just do not turn on and off synthesis of their gene product protein when they should during neurodevelopment. The specific combinations of abnormal genes that are either necessary or sufficient for the development of schizophrenia are also not known. Nevertheless, the fact that several genes linked to schizophrenia are all involved in neurodevelopment strongly indicates that in schizophrenia, something has gone wrong with the connections between neurons.

Dysconnectivity

The results of abnormal genetic programming during critical periods of neurodevelopment could include selecting the wrong neurons to survive in the fetal brain (Figure 1-54A),

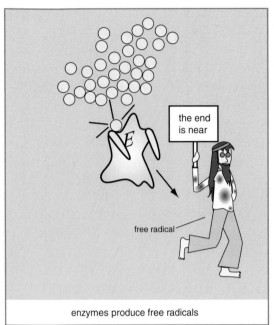

enzymes produce free radicals

FIGURE 1-49 Cellular events occurring during excitotoxicity, part 3. Once excessive glutamate causes too much calcium to enter the neuron and calcium activates dangerous enzymes, these enzymes go on to produce troublesome free radicals. Free radicals are chemicals that are capable of destroying other cellular components, such as organelles and membranes, by destructive chemical reactions.

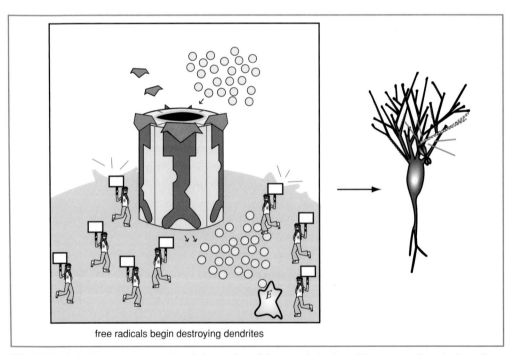

free radicals begin destroying dendrites

FIGURE 1-50 Cellular events occurring during excitotoxicity, part 4. As the calcium accumulates in the cell, and the enzymes produce more and more free radicals, they begin to destroy the dendrites that serve as postsynaptic targets of glutamate.

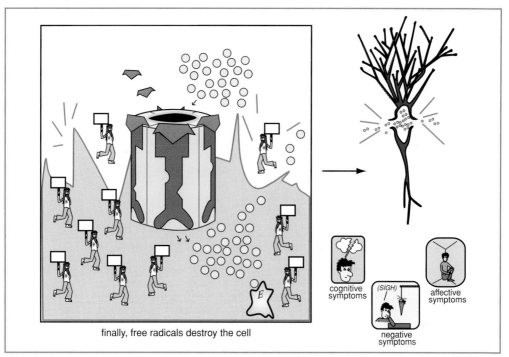

FIGURE 1-51 Cellular events occurring during excitotoxicity, part 5. Eventually, too many free radicals lead to indiscriminate destruction of various parts of the neuron, especially its neuronal and nuclear membranes and critical organelles such as energy-producing mitochondria. The damage can be so great that the free radicals essentially destroy the whole neuron. This level of destruction may be related to deficit states in schizophrenia and be associated with cognitive, negative, and affective symptoms.

having neurons migrate to the wrong places (Figure 1-54B), having neurons innervate the wrong targets, perhaps from getting the nurturing signals mixed up so that what innervates these neurons is also mixed up (Figure 1-54C), or having abnormal development of the glial cells so that they are unable to myelinate neurons properly (Figure 1-54D).

To the extent that something is wrong with major susceptibility genes for schizophrenia during the formation of the brain before birth, DISC-1 could affect early neurogenesis (Figure 1-54A), neuronal migration (Figure 1-54B) and dendritic organization (Figure 1-54C), whereas neuregulin could affect neuronal migration, especially of GABA-ergic interneurons (Figure 1-54B) as well as myelination of neurons once they have migrated into place in the forming brain (Figure 1-54D). These neurodevelopmental processes are absolutely critical for normal brain development, occur over large distances, and impact the functioning of the brain for an entire lifetime.

Abnormal synaptogenesis

Although it is possible that schizophrenia susceptibility genes may impact brain development once and forever in a type of fetal "hit and run" damage that is complete by the time the brain is formed, it is also possible that an abnormal neurodevelopmental process continues in the schizophrenic brain throughout a lifetime. Most neurons form, are selected, migrate, differentiate, and myelinate before birth, but the process of neurogenesis continues for a

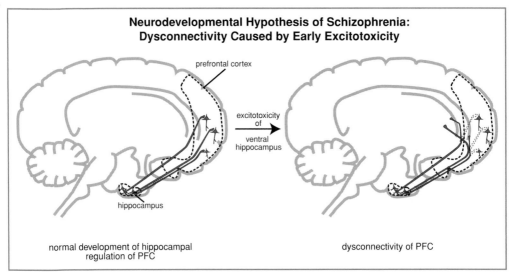

Neurodevelopmental Hypothesis of Schizophrenia: Dysconnectivity Caused by Early Excitotoxicity

prefrontal cortex

excitotoxicity of

ventral hippocampus

hippocampus

normal development of hippocampal regulation of PFC

dysconnectivity of PFC

FIGURE 1-52 **Neurodevelopmental hypothesis of schizophrenia.** Neurodevelopmental theories of schizophrenia suggest that the disorder occurs as a result of abnormalities in brain development. Excitotoxicity that occurs early in development, before the completion of synaptic connections, could result in dysconnectivity between brain regions and consequently symptoms of mental illness. For example, with normal development the ventral hippocampus forms connections with cortical pyramidal neurons to regulate activity in the prefrontal cortex (left). Excitotoxicity in the ventral hippocampus prior to completion of these connections could impact development of the prefrontal cortex, causing abnormal neuronal connections that may lead to symptoms of schizophrenia (right).

lifetime in selected brain areas. Perhaps more importantly, synaptogenesis, synaptic strengthening, elimination, and reorganization continue over a lifetime. Thus, to the extent that schizophrenia susceptibility genes affect synapse formation (Figure 1-53), they have the potential to affect ongoing brain function for a lifetime.

Many of the known susceptibility genes for schizophrenia have a profound impact on synaptogenesis (Figures 1-53 and 1-55A and B). Dysbindin, BDNF, DISC-1, and neuregulin all affect normal synapse formation; thus some combination of abnormalities in these molecules could lead to abnormal synapse formation in schizophrenia (Figure 1-55A). For example, abnormal genetic programming of dysbindin could affect synaptic cytoarchitecture and scaffolding in schizophrenia, whereas abnormal programming of DISC-1 and neuregulin could affect dendritic morphology and together lead to structurally abnormal synapses in schizophrenia (Figure 1-55B).

NMDA receptors, AMPA receptors, and synaptogenesis

Earlier in this chapter we reviewed the NMDA receptor hypofunction hypothesis of schizophrenia (illustrated in Figures 1-39 through 1-42). Supporting this hypothesis are observations that several of the known susceptibility genes for schizophrenia impact the NMDA receptor (Figures 1-55C and D and 1-56 through 1-58). Dysbindin, DISC-1, and neuregulin are all involved in the normal "strengthening" of glutamate synapses (Figure 1-55C). Normally, when glutamate synapses are active, their NMDA receptors trigger an electrical phenomenon known as long-term potentiation (LTP). With the help of dysbindin, DISC-1, and neuregulin, LTP leads to structural and functional changes of the

TABLE 1-12 Susceptibility genes for schizophrenia

Genes for:
Dysbindin (dystrobrevin binding protein 1 or DTNBP1)
Neuregulin (NRG1)
DISC1 (disrupted in schizophrenia 1)
DAOA (d-amino acid oxidase activator; G72/G30)
DAO (d-amino acid oxidase)
RGS4 (regulator of G protein signaling 4)
COMT (Catechol-O-methyl transferase)
CHRNA7 (alpha-7 nicotinic cholinergic receptor)
GAD1 (glutamic acid decarboxylase 1)
GRM3 (mGluR3)
PPP3CC
PRODH2
AKT1
ERBB4
FEZ1
MUTED
MRDS1 (OFCC1)
BDNF (brain-derived neurotrophic factor)
Nur77
MAO-A (monoamine oxidase A)
Spinophylin
Calcyon
Tyrosine hydroxylase
Dopamine-D2 receptor (D2R)
Dopamine-D3 receptor (D3R)

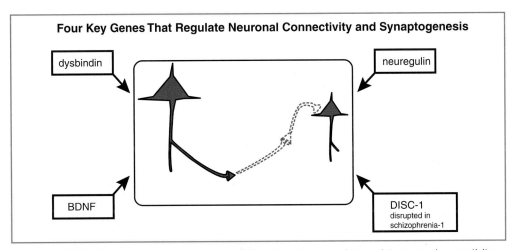

FIGURE 1-53 BDNF, dysbindin, neuregulin, and DISC-1. Four key genes that regulate neuronal connectivity and synaptogenesis in schizophrenia are the genes that code for the proteins brain derived neurotrophic factor (BDNF), dysbindin, neuregulin, and DISC-1 (disrupted in schizophrenia-1).

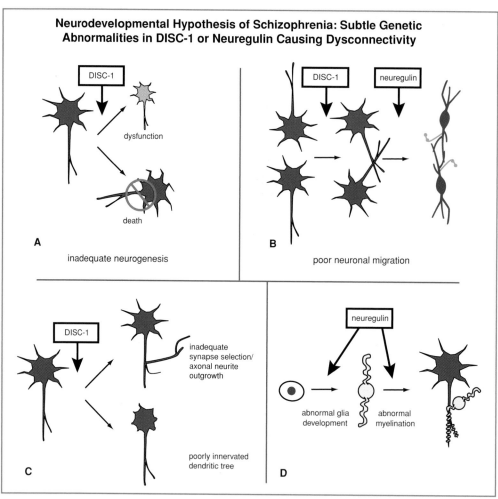

FIGURE 1-54A, B, C, and D Neurodevelopmental hypothesis of schizophrenia: subtle genetic abnormalities in DISC-1 or neuregulin causing dysconnectivity. DISC-1 (disrupted in schizophrenia-1) is a protein that is involved in neurogenesis (**A**), neuronal migration (**B**), and dendritic organization (**C**). Neuregulin is involved in neuronal migration (**B**), genesis of glial cells (**D**), and myelination of neurons by glial cells (**D**). Thus, subtle genetic abnormalities in the genes for DISC-1 or neuregulin can disrupt these processes, causing dysconnectivity among neurons, abnormal functioning of neuronal circuits among neurons linked together, increased risk of schizophrenia, and ultimately the symptoms of schizophrenia.

synapse that make neurotransmission more efficient. This includes increasing the number of AMPA receptors (Figure 1-55C).

AMPA receptors are important for mediating excitatory neurotransmission and depolarization at glutamate synapses. Thus, more AMPA receptors can mean a "strengthened" synapse (Figure 1-55C). If something is wrong with the genes that regulate synaptic strengthening, it is possible that this causes NMDA receptors to be hypoactive, leading to ineffective LTP and fewer AMPA receptors trafficking into the postsynaptic neuron. Such a synapse would be "weak," theoretically causing inefficient information processing in its circuit and thus symptoms of schizophrenia (Figure 1-55C).

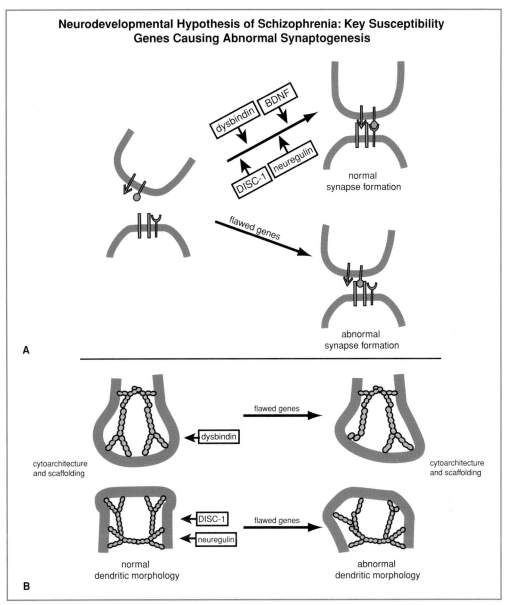

FIGURE 1-55A and B Neurodevelopmental hypothesis of schizophrenia: key susceptibility genes causing abnormal synaptogenesis, part 1. Dysbindin, brain-derived neurotrophic factor (BDNF), DISC-1 (disrupted in schizophrenia-1), and neuregulin are all involved in synapse formation. Any subtle molecular abnormalities in these genes could therefore lead to abnormal synapse formation (**A**). Specifically, abnormal genetic programming of dysbindin could affect synaptic cytoarchitecture and scaffolding, while abnormal genetic programming of DISC-1 and neuregulin could affect dendritic morphology; any of these could contribute to abnormal synapse formation and increased risk for schizophrenia (**B**).

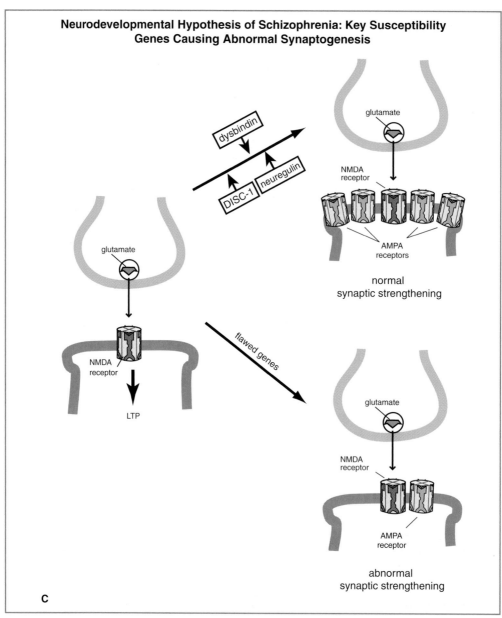

Neurodevelopmental Hypothesis of Schizophrenia: Key Susceptibility Genes Causing Abnormal Synaptogenesis

FIGURE 1-55C Neurodevelopmental hypothesis of schizophrenia: key susceptibility genes causing abnormal synaptogenesis, part 2. Dysbindin, DISC-1 (disrupted in schizophrenia-1), and neuregulin are all involved in "strengthening" of glutamate synapses. Under normal circumstances, N-methyl-d-aspartate (NMDA) receptors in active glutamate synapses trigger long-term potentiation (LTP), which leads to structural and functional changes of the synapse to make it more efficient, or "strengthened." In particular, this process leads to an increased number of alpha-amino-3-hydroxy-5-methyl-4-isoxazolepropionic acid (AMPA) receptors, which are important for mediating glutamatergic neurotransmission. If the genes that regulate strengthening of glutamate synapses are abnormal, then this could cause hypofunctioning of NMDA receptors, with a resultant decrease in LTP and fewer AMPA receptors. This would theoretically lead to increased risk of developing schizophrenia, and these abnormal synapses could mediate the symptoms of schizophrenia.

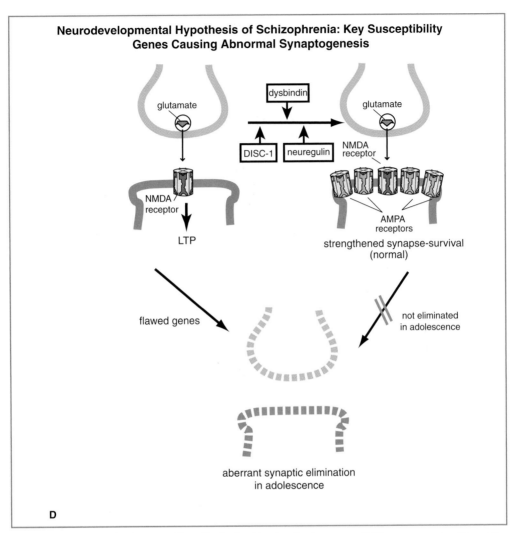

Neurodevelopmental Hypothesis of Schizophrenia: Key Susceptibility Genes Causing Abnormal Synaptogenesis

FIGURE 1-55D Neurodevelopmental hypothesis of schizophrenia: key susceptibility genes causing abnormal synaptogenesis, part 3. Strengthened synapses [for glutamate, synapses with efficient N-methyl-d-aspartate (NMDA) neurotransmission and multiple alpha-amino-3-hydroxy-5-methyl-4-isoxazolepropionic acid (AMPA) receptors] are more likely to survive than weak synapses. If the genes that regulate strengthening of glutamate synapses are abnormal, then not only might these synapses be weak but they also may be at increased risk for elimination, especially during adolescence, when there is massive restructuring of the synapses in the brain.

Furthermore, the "strength" of a synapse is likely to determine whether it is eliminated or maintained (Figure 1-55D). Specifically, "strong" synapses with efficient NMDA neurotransmission and many AMPA receptors survive, whereas "weak" synapses with few AMPA receptors may be targets for elimination (Figure 1-55D). This normally shapes the brain's circuits so that the most critical synapses are not only strengthened but also enabled to survive the selection process, keeping the most efficient and most frequently utilized synapses while eliminating those that are inefficient and rarely utilized. However, if critical synapses are not adequately strengthened in schizophrenia, it could lead to their

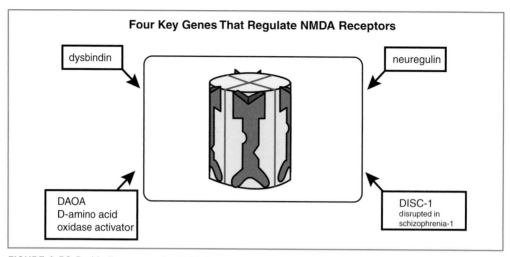

FIGURE 1-56 Dysbindin, neuregulin, DISC-1 and DAOA. Four key genes that regulate N-methyl-d-aspartate (NMDA) receptors are dysbindin, neuregulin, DISC-1 (disrupted in schizophrenia-1), and d-amino acid oxidase activator (DAOA).

elimination, disrupting information flow from circuits now deprived of synaptic connections where communication needs to be efficient (Figure 1-55D).

Competitive elimination of "weak" but critical synapses during adolescence could even explain why schizophrenia has onset at this time. Normally, almost half of the brain's synapses are eliminated in adolescence. If abnormalities in genes for dysbindin, neuregulin, and/or DISC-1 lead to the failure of critical synapses to be strengthened, these critical synapses may be mistakenly eliminated during adolescence, with disastrous consequences – namely, the onset of symptoms of schizophrenia.

It is possible that "the die is cast" much earlier, due to aberrant neuronal selection, migration, and connections that remain silent until adolescence. However, in the late teens to twenties, abnormal synaptic restructuring due to elimination of necessary synapses that are not adequately strengthened could unmask neurodevelopmental problems that were previously hidden. To add insult to injury, ongoing problems in synaptic strengthening throughout adulthood in a schizophrenic patient may lead to perpetual elimination of critical synapses, causing the formation of new symptoms or exacerbation of ongoing symptoms due to circuits with progressively and unremittingly aberrant synaptogenesis.

Convergence of susceptibility genes for schizophrenia upon glutamate synapses

Many of the known susceptibility genes for schizophrenia (Table 1-12) regulate not only synaptogenesis at glutamate synapses (Figure 1-53), but also many other functions linked to glutamate neurotransmission, such as the NMDA receptor (Figure 1-56).

For example, the gene for DAOA (d-amino acid oxidase activator) codes for a protein that activates the enzyme DAO (d-amino acid oxidase) (Figures 1-56 and 1-57). We have previously discussed how DAO degrades the cotransmitter d-serine, which acts at glutamate synapses and at NMDA receptors (Figure 1-35). DAOA activates this enzyme (Figure 1-57A); therefore abnormalities in the gene for DAOA would be expected to alter the metabolism of d-serine. This, in turn, would alter glutamate neurotransmission at NMDA receptors (Figure 1-57A).

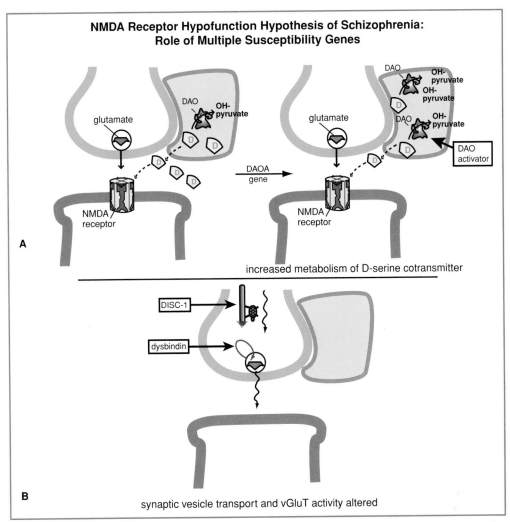

FIGURE 1-57A and B NMDA receptor hypofunction hypothesis of schizophrenia: role of multiple susceptibility genes, part 1. (A) d-amino acid oxidase activator (DAOA) is a protein that activates the enzyme d-amino acid oxidase (DAO). DAO converts d-serine into OH-pyruvate (on the left). Thus, abnormalities in the gene for DAOA could lead to abnormal functioning of the enzyme DAO, and this would change the metabolism of d-serine. Changes in the availability of d-serine would affect glutamate neurotransmission at N-methyl-d-aspartate (NMDA) receptors. If DAO activity were increased and d-serine levels thus decreased, this would lead to hypofunctioning of NMDA receptors (on the right). Thus, an abnormality in the gene for DAOA could increase risk for schizophrenia by altering the function of NMDA receptors. **(B)** Abnormalities in dysbindin and DISC-1 (disrupted in schizophrenia-1) could lead to alterations in the transport of synaptic vesicles into the presynaptic nerve terminal and could also lead to changes in the vesicular transport of glutamate by the glutamate transporter (vGluT). Both would be predicted to cause changes in the presynaptic storage of glutamate, and these could alter the function of NMDA receptors during glutamate neurotransmission. Thus, abnormalities in dysbindin and/or DISC-1 could lead to hypofunctioning of NMDA receptors and increase the risk for schizophrenia.

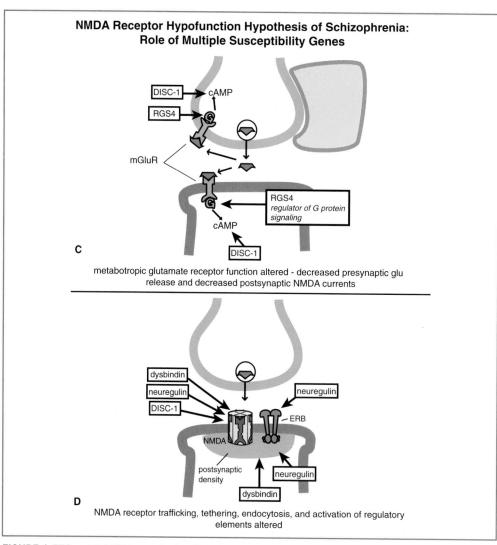

NMDA Receptor Hypofunction Hypothesis of Schizophrenia: Role of Multiple Susceptibility Genes

C

metabotropic glutamate receptor function altered - decreased presynaptic glu release and decreased postsynaptic NMDA currents

D

NMDA receptor trafficking, tethering, endocytosis, and activation of regulatory elements altered

FIGURE 1-57C and D NMDA receptor hypofunction hypothesis of schizophrenia: role of multiple susceptibility genes, part 2. (**C**) Abnormalities in the genes for DISC-1 (disrupted in schizophrenia-1) could lead to disruptions of cyclic adenosine monophosphate (cAMP) signaling and consequently to alterations in the functioning of metabotropic glutamate receptors. Abnormalities in the gene that codes for the regulator of G protein signaling (RGS4) could also alter metabotropic glutamate receptor signaling. These changes would alter glutamate neurotransmission by decreasing the release of presynaptic glutamate, thus leading to a decrease in postsynaptic N-methyl-d-aspartate (NMDA) currents. Together, this would cause NMDA receptor hypofunctioning, which could increase the risk for schizophrenia. (**D**) Abnormalities in dysbindin, neuregulin, and/or DISC-1 could lead to alterations in NMDA receptor trafficking, tethering, endocytosis, and activation of postsynaptic regulatory elements. That would cause NMDA receptor hypofunctioning and could increase the risk for developing schizophrenia.

Dysbindin regulates the activity of vGluT, the vesicular transporter for glutamate (Figure 1-57B). DISC-1 affects the transport of synaptic vesicles into presynaptic glutamate nerve terminals (Figure 1-57B) and also regulates cAMP signaling, which would affect the functions of glutamate neurotransmission mediated by metabotropic glutamate receptors (Figure 1-57C). Another schizophrenia susceptibility gene is RGS4 (regulator of G protein signaling) (Table 1-12), and this gene product also impacts metabotropic glutamate receptor signaling through the G protein – coupled signal transduction system (Figure 1-57C).

Finally, numerous susceptibility genes regulate various elements of NMDA receptor – mediated signaling (Figure 1-57D). Dysbindin, neuregulin, and DISC-1 all affect NMDA receptor number by altering NMDA receptor trafficking to the postsynaptic membrane, NMDA receptor tethering within that membrane, and NMDA receptor endocytosis, which cycles receptors out of the postsynaptic membrane to remove them (Figure 1-57D). Both dysbindin and neuregulin affect the formation and function of the postsynaptic density, a set of proteins that interact with the postsynaptic membrane to provide both structural and functional regulatory elements for neurotransmission and for NMDA receptors (Figure 1-57D). Neuregulin also activates an ERB signaling system that is colocalized with NMDA receptors (Figure 1-57D). This signaling system is a member of the receptor tyrosine kinase and neurotrophin signal transduction system. These ERB receptors also interact with the postsynaptic density and may be involved in mediating the neuroplasticity triggered by NMDA receptors (Figure 1-57D).

Thus, there is a powerful convergence of the known susceptibility genes for schizophrenia upon connectivity, synaptogenesis, and neurotransmission at glutamate synapses and specifically at NMDA receptors (Figures 1-55C and D, 1-56, 1-57, and 1-58). These observations strongly support the hypothesis of NMDA receptor hypofunction as a plausible theory for schizophrenia. Genes that code for any number of subtle molecular abnormalities linked to NMDA receptor function in specific brain circuits theoretically create inefficient information processing at glutamate synapses, which can produce the symptoms of schizophrenia. If enough of these genetically mediated abnormalities occur simultaneously in a permissive environment, the syndrome of schizophrenia could be the result.

What are the candidate susceptibility genes for schizophrenia and how do they affect the NMDA receptor? Several of these are listed in Table 1-12 and many are shown in Figure 1-58. Clearly, numerous susceptibility genes can affect glutamate and its cotransmitter d-serine directly (e.g., DISC-1, neuregulin, dysbindin, DAOA, RGS4); their hypothesized actions on the glutamate system are illustrated in Figures 1-53 through 1-58. In addition, a number of other neurotransmitters such as dopamine, serotonin, GABA, and acetylcholine also affect the NMDA receptor, not only by direct interaction with glutamate neurons via brain circuits that utilize these other neurotransmitters but also by virtue of the fact that several of the genes that affect glutamate (e.g., neuregulin, RGS4) also affect these other neurotransmitters (Figure 1-58). Additional susceptibility genes may modulate these other neurotransmitter systems, leading to their aberrant modulation of NMDA plasticity and thus contributing to the genetic risk for schizophrenia. Some of these other genes regulate the receptors, enzymes, signaling molecules, and synapses for serotonin, dopamine, and acetylcholine (Table 1-12 and Figure 1-58). With sufficient combinations of directly and indirectly acting genetic influences, the NMDA receptor may not function properly, become hypofunctional, and – in addition to causing the changes in neuronal activity within brain circuits already described (see Figures 1-39 through 1-42) – also cause abnormal

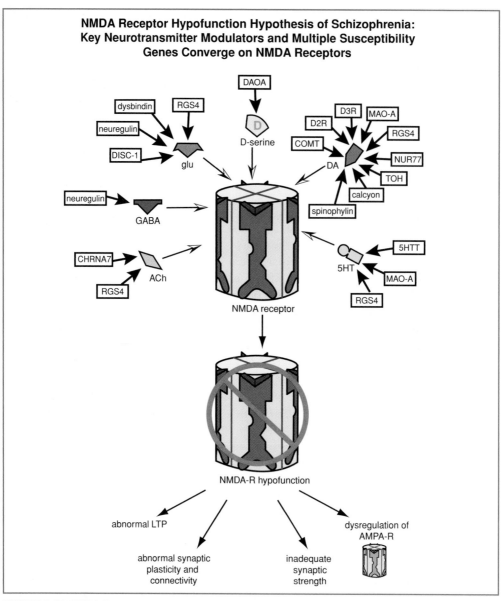

FIGURE 1-58 NMDA (N-methyl-d-aspartate) receptor hypofunction hypothesis of schizophrenia: key neurotransmitter modulators and multiple susceptibility genes converge on NMDA receptors. There is a powerful convergence of susceptibility genes for schizophrenia upon the connectivity, synaptogenesis, and neurotransmission at glutamate synapses and specifically at NMDA receptors, supporting the NMDA receptor hypofunction hypothesis of schizophrenia. The specific hypothesized actions of four key genes shown here are illustrated in detail in Figure 1-57 [i.e., the susceptibility genes DAOA (d-amino acid oxidase activator), dysbindin, neuregulin, and DISC-1 (disrupted in schizophrenia-1)]. Additional susceptibility genes are also shown here, including those that affect various neurotransmitters involved in modulating glutamate and NMDA receptors, namely gamma-aminobutyric acid (GABA), acetylcholine (ACh), dopamine (DA) and serotonin (5HT). That is, abnormalities in genes for various neurotransmitters that regulate NMDA receptors could have additional downstream actions on glutamate functioning at NMDA receptors. Thus, genes that regulate these other neurotransmitters may also constitute susceptibility genes for schizophrenia. This includes genes that affect ACh, such as the genes for RGS4 (regulator of G protein signaling 4) and for CHRNA7 (the alpha-7 nicotinic cholinergic receptor subtype); genes that affect 5HT (RGS4 as well as the genes for the monoamine oxidase A,

long-term potentiation, abnormal synaptic plasticity and connectivity, dysregulation of AMPA receptors, and inadequate synaptic strength with those circuits (Figure 1-58).

The bottom line

Genetics studies in schizophrenia have identified a number of susceptibility genes that increase risk for schizophrenia but do not cause schizophrenia. Since the best-understood and most replicated of these genes are involved in neurodevelopment, neuronal connectivity, and synaptogenesis, most scientists now believe that schizophrenia is caused by various possible combinations of many different genes plus stressors from the environment conspiring to cause abnormal neurodevelopment. Genetic and pharmacological evidence in schizophrenia also points to abnormal neurotransmission at glutamate synapses, possibly involving hypofunctional NMDA receptors. Several new therapies that target NMDA receptors are being tested, and new treatments for schizophrenia are discussed in Chapter 2.

Neuroimaging circuits in schizophrenia

Functional imaging of circuits in patients with schizophrenia suggests that information processing is abnormal in key brain areas linked to specific symptoms of this disorder. For example, schizophrenia is characterized by cognitive symptoms that are theoretically linked to information processing by circuits that involve the dorsolateral prefrontal cortex (DLPFC). The n-back test (Figure 1-59A) can be used to activate the DLPFC (Figure 1-59B).

Some studies show that activation of the prefrontal cortex is low in schizophrenia, but other studies show that it is high (Figure 1-60). The best explanation for this may be that prefrontal cortical dysfunction in schizophrenia is likely to be more complicated than just "up" (hyperactivation) or "down" (hypoactivation) but might be better characterized as "out of tune." According to this concept, either too much or too little activation of neuronal activity in the prefrontal cortex is suboptimal and can potentially be symptomatic.

How can circuits in schizophrenia be both hyper- and hypoactive? Schizophrenic patients appear to utilize greater prefrontal resources in performing cognitive tasks and yet achieve lower accuracy because they have cognitive impairment despite their best efforts. To perform near normally, schizophrenic patients engage the DLPFC, but they do so inefficiently, recruiting greater neural resources and hyperactivating the DLPFC (Figure 1-60). When they are performing poorly, schizophrenic patients do not appropriately engage and sustain the DLPFC and thus show hypoactivation (Figure 1-60). Thus, DLPFC circuits in schizophrenic patients can either be underactive and hypofrontal or overactive and inefficient.

FIGURE 1-58 *(Cont.)* or MAO-A); and the genes for the serotonin transporter (5HTT); finally, multiple genes that affect DA (RGS4, MAO-A), and also genes for the enzymes catechol-O-methyl-transferase (COMT) and tyrosine hydroxylase (TOH); genes for the D2- and D3-dopamine receptors (D2R and D3R), and finally genes for the regulatory proteins spinophylin and calcyon. The idea is that any of these susceptibility genes could conspire to cause NMDA receptor hypofunction, which would lead to abnormal long-term potentiation (LTP), abnormal synaptic plasticity and connectivity, inadequate synaptic strength, and/or dysregulation of alpha-amino-3-hydroxy-5-methyl-4-isoxazolepropionic acid (AMPA) receptors. Any combination of sufficient genetic risk factors with sufficient stress or environmental risk will result in the susceptibility for schizophrenia to become manifest as the disease of schizophrenia with the presence of full syndrome symptoms.

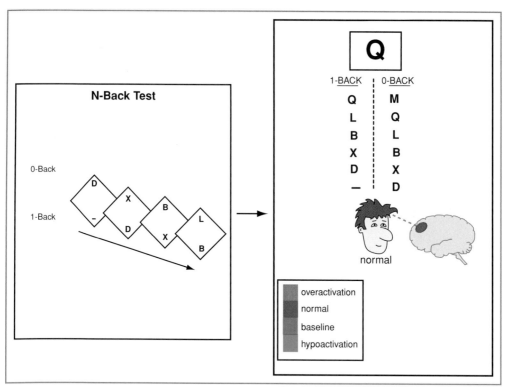

FIGURE 1-59 n-back test. Functional neuroimaging studies have suggested that information processing in schizophrenia is abnormal in certain brain regions. Information processing during cognitive tasks has been evaluated using the n-back test. In the 0-back variant of the test, participants view a number on a screen and then indicate what the number was. In the 1-back test, participants are shown a stimulus but do not respond; after viewing the second stimulus, the participant then pushes a button corresponding to the first stimulus. The "n" can be any number, with higher numbers associated with greater difficulty. Performing the n-back test results in activation of the dorsolateral prefrontal cortex (DLPFC), shown here by the DLPFC lit up as purple (normal activation). The degree of activation indicates how efficient the information processing is in DLPFC, with both overactivation and hypoactivation associated with inefficient information processing.

It is interesting to note that unaffected siblings of patients with schizophrenia may have the very same inefficient information processing in DLPFC that schizophrenic patients have (Figure 1-61). Although such unaffected siblings might have a mild degree of cognitive impairment, they do not share the full clinical phenotype of the syndrome of schizophrenia; however, neuroimaging reveals that they may share the same biological endophenotype of inefficient DLPFC functioning while performing cognitive tasks that characterizes their schizophrenic siblings (Figure 1-61). The unaffected siblings of a schizophrenic patient may thus share some of the susceptibility genes for schizophrenia with their affected sibling but not enough of these risk genes to have the full syndrome of schizophrenia itself. Functional neuroimaging has the potential of unmasking clinically silent biological endophenotypes in the unaffected siblings of schizophrenic patients who share some of the same risk genes, but do not have sufficient combinations of risk genes to develop the illness of schizophrenia. Functional neuroimaging also has the potential of unmasking clinically silent biological endophenotypes in presymptomatic patients destined to progress to the full schizophrenia syndrome. However, much further research is required to see if this will become clinically useful.

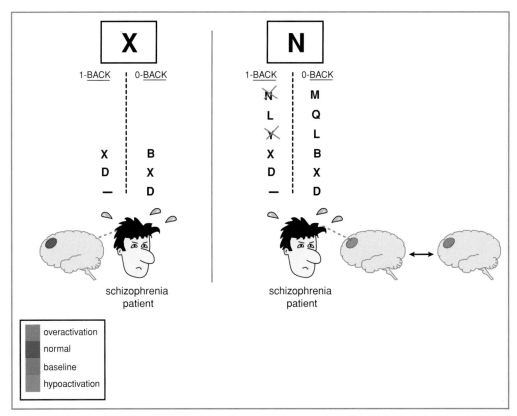

FIGURE 1-60 n-back test in schizophrenia. Patients with schizophrenia exhibit inefficient information processing during cognitive challenges such as the n-back test. To perform near normal, these individuals must recruit greater neuronal resources, resulting in hyperactivation of the dorsolateral prefrontal cortex (DLPFC). Under increased cognitive load, however, schizophrenic patients do not appropriately engage and sustain the DLPFC, with resultant hypoactivation.

Affective and negative symptoms of schizophrenia may involve other areas of the prefrontal cortex, such as orbital, medial, and ventral areas (see Figure 1-14). These brain areas, along with the amygdala, nucleus accumbens, and other regions, comprise a "ventral" system involved in emotional processing. This ventral system interacts with a "dorsal" system that includes the DLPFC and modulates the output from the ventral system (Figure 1-62).

The ventral system (Figure 1-62) includes orbital, ventral, and medial areas of prefrontal cortex (shown in Figure 1-14), amygdala (shown in Figure 1-63), and nucleus accumbens (shown in Figure 1-62) – brain regions that are all important for the identification and appraisal of emotional stimuli and for generating an appropriate emotional response. The dorsal system includes not just the DLPFC but also the hippocampus. This system marshals the cognitive resources necessary either to maintain the emotional response from the ventral system or to modulate it. The dorsal system selects an appropriate behavioral output in response not only to emotions but also to demands from the environment and from the individual's internal goals.

Schizophrenia has long been recognized as having impairments in the ability to identify and accurately interpret emotions from overt sources, including facial expressions. This may

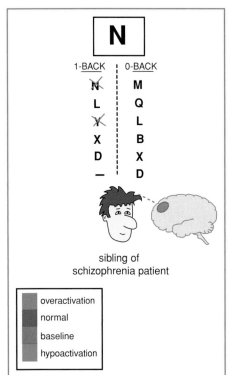

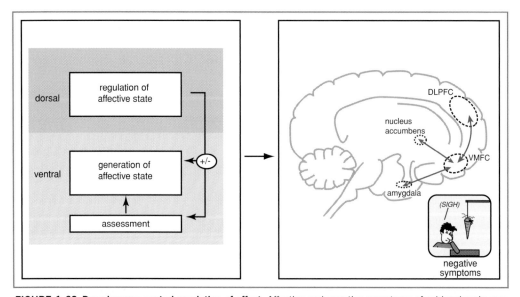

FIGURE 1-62 Dorsal versus ventral regulation of affect. Affective and negative symptoms of schizophrenia may
be generated by a ventral system that includes the ventromedial prefrontal cortex (VMFC), nucleus accumbens,
and amygdala and regulated by a dorsal system that includes the dorsolateral prefrontal cortex (DLPFC).

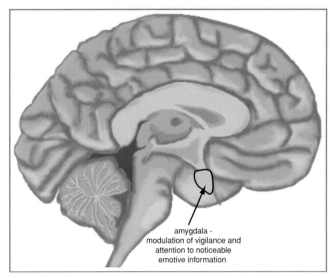

FIGURE 1-63 Amygdala. The amygdala is involved in modulation of vigilance, attention, and reactions to noticeable emotive information. Functional neuroimaging studies have examined activity in the amygdala to determine the efficiency of information processing in schizophrenic patients during exposure to emotional stimuli.

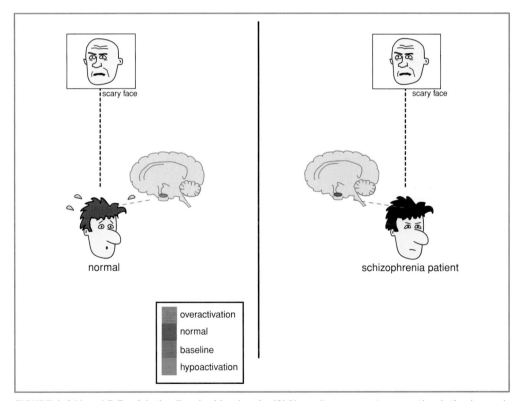

FIGURE 1-64A and B Fearful stimuli and schizophrenia. (A) Normally, exposure to an emotional stimulus, such as a scary face, causes hyperactivation in the amygdala. **(B)** Schizophrenic patients often have impairments in the ability to identify and interpret emotional stimuli. The underlying neurobiological explanation for this may be inefficient information processing within the ventral system. In this example, the amygdala is not appropriately engaged during exposure to an emotional stimulus.

be due to inefficient information processing within the ventral system and can be measured by imaging the response of the amygdala (Figure 1-63) to emotional input, especially from facial expressions. The amygdala is normally activated by looking at scary, threatening faces or by assessing how happy or sad a face may be and while attempting to match the emotions of one face to another (Figure 1-64A).

Whereas normals may activate the amygdala in response to scary or fearful or emotionally charged faces (Figure 1-64A), patients with schizophrenia may not (Figure 1-64B). This may represent distortion of reality as well as an impairment in recognizing negative emotions and in decoding negative emotions in schizophrenia. Failure to mount the "normal" emotional response to a scary face can also represent an inability to interpret social cues and may lead to distortions in judgment and reasoning in schizophrenia. Thus, these negative and affective symptoms of schizophrenia may be due in part to lack of emotional processing under circumstances when this should be occurring.

On the other hand, a neutral face or neutral stimulus may provoke little activation of the amygdala in a normal person (Figure 1-65A), yet an overreaction in a schizophrenic patient, who may mistakenly judge people negatively or conclude wrongly that another holds strong unfavorable impressions of him or her or may even be threatening (Figure 1-65B). The activation of emotional processing in the amygdala when it is inappropriate may accompany the symptom of paranoia and lead to impaired interpersonal functioning, including problems

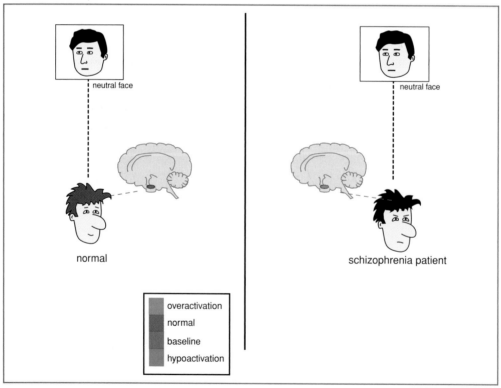

FIGURE 1-65A and B Neutral stimuli and schizophrenia. (A) Normally, exposure to a neutral stimulus, such as a neutral face, causes little activation of the amygdala. **(B)** Schizophrenic patients may mistakenly judge others as threatening, with associated inappropriate hyperactivation of the amygdala.

in social communication. Thus, schizophrenic patients may exhibit deficits in recognizing emotions, which may become manifest as either positive or negative symptoms of this disorder. The underlying biological endophenotype of amygdala activation (or lack of it) in the ventral emotional processing circuitry can be assessed with neuroimaging, whether the patient is experiencing these symptoms or not. Looking at the efficiency of emotional information processing may help clinicians identify and understand emotional symptoms that are difficult for schizophrenic patients to express.

Summary

This chapter has provided a clinical description of psychosis, with special emphasis on the psychotic illness schizophrenia. We have explained the dopamine hypothesis of schizophrenia, and the related NMDA receptor hypofunction hypothesis of schizophrenia, which are the major hypotheses for explaining the mechanism underlying positive, negative, cognitive, and affective symptoms of schizophrenia.

The major dopamine and glutamate pathways in the brain have been described. Overactivity of the mesolimbic dopamine system may mediate the positive symptoms of psychosis and may be linked to hypofunctioning NMDA glutamate receptors in the descending corticobrainstem glutamate pathway. Underactivity of the mesocortical dopamine system may mediate the negative, cognitive, and affective symptoms of schizophrenia and could also be linked to hypofunctioning NMDA receptors.

The synthesis, metabolism, reuptake, and receptors for both dopamine and glutamate have been described above. Dopamine-2 receptors are targets of all known antipsychotic drugs. NMDA glutamate receptors require interaction not only with the neurotransmitter glutamate but also with the cotransmitters glycine or d-serine.

Both the neurodegenerative hypothesis and the neurodevelopmental hypothesis of schizophrenia have been discussed. Although neurodegenerative events such as fetal brain insults or excitotoxicity may contribute to schizophrenia, current research points most strongly to a neurodevelopmental basis, mediated by a whole host of susceptibility genes that regulate neuronal connectivity and synapse formation. A great deal of genetic research converges on the possibility that abnormal formation of synapses – particularly those that utilize glutamate as neurotransmitter and those that function with NMDA receptors – is a central biological flaw in schizophrenia.

Malfunctioning neural circuits can be imaged in schizophrenic patients, including those in the dorsolateral prefrontal cortex linked to cognitive symptoms and those in the amygdala linked to symptoms of emotional dysregulation.

Antipsychotic Agents

This chapter explores antipsychotic drugs with an emphasis on treatments for schizophrenia. These treatments include not only conventional antipsychotic drugs but also the newer atypical antipsychotic drugs, which have largely replaced the older conventional agents in many countries. Atypical antipsychotics are also used as mood stabilizers for the manic, depressed, and maintenance phases of bipolar disorder in both adults and in children. Atypical antipsychotics have many other "off-label" uses, from augmentation of antidepressants in treatment-resistant depression and of anxiolytics in treatment-resistant anxiety disorders to treatment of psychosis and behavioral disturbances in Alzheimer's disease and other dementias. Here we will discuss the use of conventional and atypical antipsychotics for the treatment of schizophrenia and also take a look into the future by discussing numerous new drugs under development for schizophrenia.

Antipsychotic drugs exhibit possibly the most complex pharmacological mechanisms of any drug class in the field of clinical psychopharmacology. To assist the reader in mastering this critical area of therapeutics in psychopharmacology, we have organized this chapter into five sections: first, the classic conventional antipsychotics; second, the contrasting pharmacological properties that make an antipsychotic atypical; third, a discussion of the multiple receptor actions of antipsychotics as well as their pharmacokinetics, comparing and contrasting the properties of the various individual atypical antipsychotics; fourth, a practical analysis of how these agents are put to use in clinical practice; and fifth, a discussion of new therapeutics for schizophrenia currently in development.

The reader is referred to standard reference manuals and textbooks for practical prescribing information, such as drug doses, because this chapter emphasizes basic pharmacological concepts regarding mechanisms of action and not practical issues such as how to prescribe these drugs (for that information, see, for example, S. M. Stahl, *Essential Psychopharmacology: The Prescriber's Guide*, which is a companion to this book). The pharmacological concepts developed here should, however, help the reader understand the rationale for how to use antipsychotic agents based on their interactions with different neurotransmitter systems. Such interactions can often explain both the therapeutic actions and the side effects of antipsychotic medications and thus can provide very helpful background information for prescribers of these therapeutic agents.

What makes an antipsychotic conventional?

In this section we will discuss the pharmacological properties of the first drugs that were proven to treat schizophrenia effectively. These drugs are usually called conventional antipsychotics, but they are sometimes also called classic or "typical" antipsychotics. The earliest effective treatments for schizophrenia and other psychotic illnesses arose from serendipitous clinical observations more than 50 years ago, rather than from scientific knowledge of the neurobiologic basis of psychosis or of the mechanism of action of effective antipsychotic agents. Thus, the first antipsychotic drugs were discovered by accident in the 1950s, when a drug with antihistamine properties (chlorpromazine) was observed to have antipsychotic effects when tested in schizophrenic patients. Chlorpromazine indeed has antihistaminic activity, but its therapeutic actions in schizophrenia are not mediated by this property. Once chlorpromazine was observed to be an effective antipsychotic agent, it was tested experimentally to uncover its mechanism of antipsychotic action.

Early in the testing process, chlorpromazine and other antipsychotic agents were all found to cause "neurolepsis," an extreme form of slowness or absence of motor movements as well as behavioral indifference in experimental animals. The original antipsychotics were

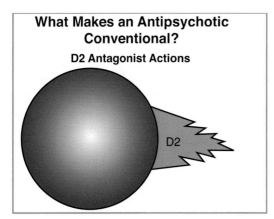

What Makes an Antipsychotic Conventional?

D2 Antagonist Actions

D2

FIGURE 2-1 D2 antagonist. Conventional antipsychotics, also called first-generation antipsychotics or typical antipsychotics, share the primary pharmacological property of D2 antagonism, which is responsible not only for their antipsychotic efficacy but also for many of their side effects. Shown here is an icon representing this single pharmacological action.

first discovered largely by their ability to produce this effect in experimental animals and are thus sometimes called "neuroleptics." A human counterpart of neurolepsis is also caused by these original (i.e., conventional) antipsychotic drugs and is characterized by psychomotor slowing, emotional quieting, and affective indifference.

D2-receptor antagonism makes an antipsychotic conventional

By the 1970s, it was widely recognized that the key pharmacological property of all neuroleptics with antipsychotic properties was their ability to block dopamine-2 (D2) receptors (Figure 2-1). This action has proven to be responsible not only for the antipsychotic efficacy of conventional antipsychotic drugs but also for most of their undesirable side effects, including neurolepsis.

The therapeutic actions of conventional antipsychotic drugs are due to blockade of D2 receptors, specifically in the mesolimbic dopamine pathway (Figure 2-2). This has the effect of reducing the hyperactivity in this pathway, which is postulated to cause the positive symptoms of psychosis, as discussed in Chapter 1 (see Figures 1-25 and 1-26). All conventional antipsychotics reduce positive psychotic symptoms about equally in schizophrenic patients studied in large multicenter trials. That is not to say that one individual patient might not occasionally respond better to one conventional antipsychotic agent than another, but there is no consistent difference in antipsychotic efficacy among the conventional antipsychotic agents. A list of many conventional antipsychotic drugs is given in Table 2-1.

Unfortunately it is not possible to block just these D2 receptors in the mesolimbic DA pathway with conventional antipsychotics because antipsychotic drugs are delivered throughout the entire brain after oral ingestion. Thus, conventional antipsychotics will seek out every D2 receptor throughout the brain and block them all (see Figures 2-3 through 2-7). This leads to a high "cost of doing business" in order to get the mesolimbic D2 receptors blocked for the treatment of positive symptoms.

Neurolepsis

D2 receptors in the mesolimbic dopamine system are postulated to mediate not only the positive symptoms of psychosis but also the normal reward system of the brain, and the nucleus accumbens is widely considered to be the "pleasure center" of the brain. It may be the final common pathway of all reward and reinforcement, including not only normal

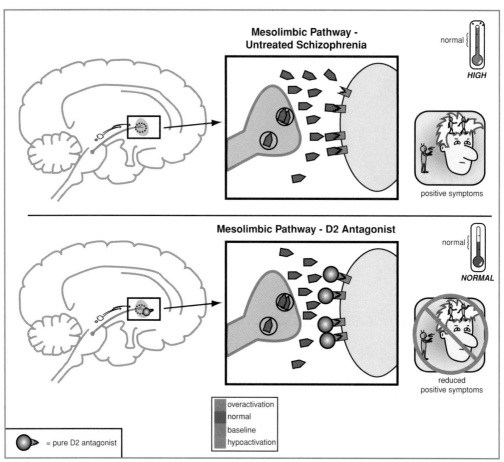

FIGURE 2-2 Mesolimbic dopamine pathway and D2 antagonists. In untreated schizophrenia, the mesolimbic dopamine pathway is hypothesized to be hyperactive, indicated here by the pathway appearing red as well as by the excess dopamine in the synapse. This leads to positive symptoms such as delusions and hallucinations. Administration of a D2 antagonist, such as a conventional antipsychotic, blocks dopamine from binding to the D2 receptor, which reduces hyperactivity in this pathway and thereby reduces positive symptoms as well.

reward (such as the pleasure of eating good food, orgasm, listening to music) but also the artificial reward of substance abuse. If D2 receptors are stimulated in some parts of the mesolimbic pathway, this can lead to the experience of pleasure. Thus if D2 receptors in the mesolimbic system are blocked, this may not only reduce positive symptoms but also block reward mechanisms, leaving patients apathetic, anhedonic, lacking motivation, and with reduced interest and joy from social interactions – a state very similar to that due to the negative symptoms of psychosis and sometimes called secondary negative symptoms.

Antipsychotics also block D2 receptors in the mesocortical DA pathway (Figure 2-3), where DA may already be deficient in schizophrenia (see Figures 1-27 through 1-29). This can cause or worsen negative and cognitive symptoms. However, since the density of D2 receptors in the cortex is much lower than in other brain areas, the lack of pleasure and negative symptoms produced by antipsychotic drugs may be more closely linked to profound blockade of D2 receptors in the mesolimbic dopamine system than to blockade of D2 receptors in the mesocortical dopamine system. An adverse behavioral state can be produced by conventional antipsychotics and is sometimes called the "neuroleptic-induced deficit

TABLE 2-1 Some conventional antipsychotics still in use

Generic Name	Trade Name
chlorpromazine	Thorazine
cyamemazine	Tercian
flupenthixol	Depixol
fluphenazine	Prolixin
haloperidol	Haldol
loxapine	Loxitane
mesoridazine	Serentil
molindone	Moban
perphenazine	Trilafon
pimozide	Orap
pipothiazine	Piportil
sulpiride	Dolmatil
thioridazine	Mellaril
thiothixene	Navane
trifluoperazine	Stelazine
zuclopenthixol	Clopixol

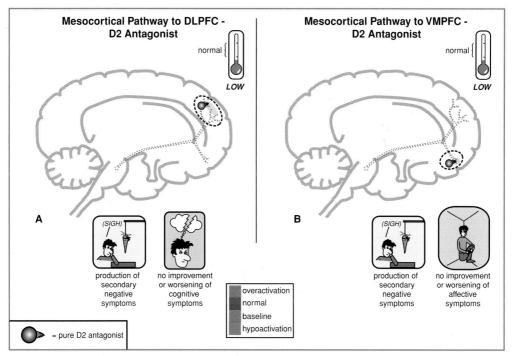

FIGURE 2-3 Mesocortical dopamine pathway and D2 antagonists. In untreated schizophrenia, the mesocortical dopamine pathways to dorsolateral prefrontal cortex (DLPFC) and to ventromedial prefrontal cortex (VMPFC) are hypothesized to be hypoactive, indicated here by the pathways appearing blue. This hypoactivity is related to cognitive symptoms (in the DLPFC), negative symptoms (in the DLPFC and VMPFC), and affective symptoms of schizophrenia (in the VMPFC). Administration of a D2 antagonist could further reduce activity in this pathway and thus not only not improve such symptoms but actually potentially worsen them.

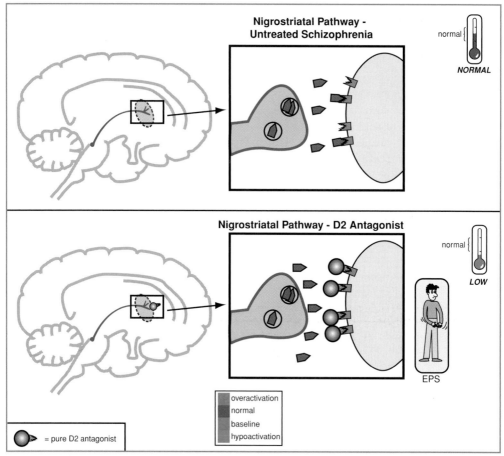

FIGURE 2-4 Nigrostriatal dopamine pathway and D2 antagonists. The nigrostriatal dopamine pathway is theoretically unaffected in untreated schizophrenia, illustrated here by the purple hue of the pathway. However, blockade of D2 receptors, as with a conventional antipsychotic, prevents dopamine from binding there and can cause motor side effects that are often collectively termed extrapyramidal symptoms (EPS).

syndrome" because it looks so much like the negative symptoms produced by schizophrenia itself and is reminiscent of neurolepsis in animals.

Extrapyramidal symptoms (EPS) and tardive dyskinesia

When D2 receptors are blocked in the nigrostriatal DA pathway, it produces disorders of movement that can appear very much like those of Parkinson's disease; that is why this is sometimes called drug-induced parkinsonism (Figure 2-4). Since the nigrostriatal pathway is part of the extrapyramidal nervous system, these motor side effects associated with blocking D2 receptors in this part of the brain are sometimes also called extrapyramidal symptoms, or EPS.

Worse yet, if these D2 receptors in the nigrostriatal DA pathway are blocked chronically (Figure 2-5), they can produce a hyperkinetic movement disorder known as tardive dyskinesia. This causes facial and tongue movements, like constant chewing, tongue protrusions, and facial grimacing as well as limb movements that can be quick, jerky, or choreiform ("dancing"). Tardive dyskinesia is thus caused by long-term administration of conventional

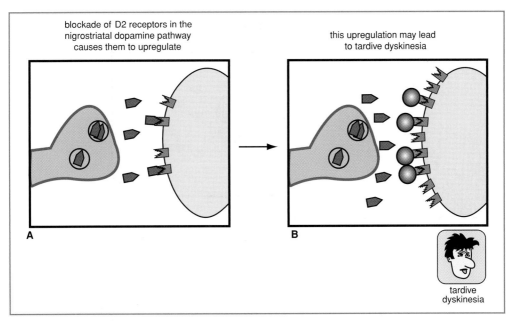

FIGURE 2-5 Tardive dyskinesia. Long-term blockade of D2 receptors in the nigrostriatal dopamine pathway can cause upregulation of those receptors, which may lead to a hyperkinetic motor condition known as tardive dyskinesia, characterized by facial and tongue movements (e.g., tongue protrusions, facial grimaces, chewing) as well as quick, jerky limb movements. This upregulation may be the consequence of the neuron's futile attempt to overcome drug-induced blockade of its dopamine receptors.

antipsychotics and is thought to be mediated by changes, sometimes irreversible, in the D2 receptors of the nigrostriatal DA pathway. Specifically, these receptors are hypothesized to become supersensitive or to "upregulate" (i.e., increase in number), perhaps in a futile attempt to overcome drug-induced blockade of these receptors (Figure 2-5).

About 5 percent of patients maintained on conventional antipsychotics will develop tardive dyskinesia every year (i.e., about 25 percent of patients by 5 years) – not a very encouraging prospect for a lifelong illness starting in the early twenties. The risk of developing tardive dyskinesia in elderly subjects may be as high as 25 percent within the first year of exposure to conventional antipsychotics. Thus, the number of patients that a psychopharmacologist needs to treat in order to harm 1 patient with tardive dyskinesia may be only 4 young patients over 5 years of conventional antipsychotic treatment or only 4 elderly patients over 1 year of conventional antipsychotic treatment. Statisticians sometimes call this the "number needed to harm."

If the D2 receptor blockade is removed early enough, tardive dyskinesia may reverse. This reversal is theoretically due to a "resetting" of these receptors by an appropriate decrease in the number or sensitivity of D2 receptors in the nigrostriatal pathway once the drug that had been blocking these receptors is removed. However, after long-term treatment, the D2 receptors apparently cannot or do not reset back to normal, even when conventional antipsychotic drugs are discontinued. This leads to irreversible tardive dyskinesia, which continues whether conventional antipsychotic drugs are administered or not.

Is there any way to predict those who will be harmed with the development of tardive dyskinesia after chronic treatment with conventional antipsychotics? Patients who develop

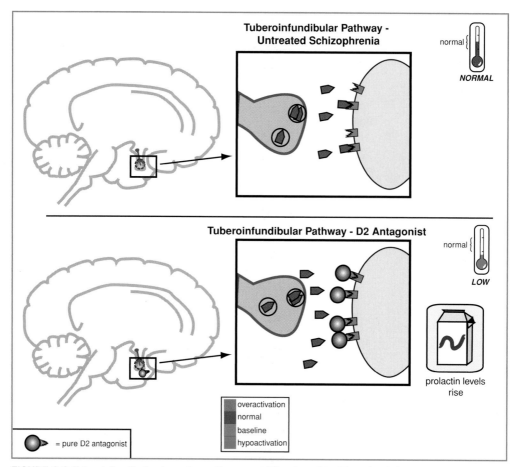

FIGURE 2-6 Tuberoinfundibular dopamine pathway and D2 antagonists. The tuberoinfundibular dopamine pathway, which projects from the hypothalamus to the pituitary gland, is theoretically "normal" in untreated schizophrenia. D2 antagonists reduce activity in this pathway by preventing dopamine from binding to D2 receptors. This causes prolactin levels to rise, which is associated with side effects such as galactorrhea (breast secretions) and amenorrhea (irregular menstrual periods).

FIGURE 2-7 Integrated theory of schizophrenia and D2 antagonists. In untreated schizophrenia, dopamine output is high in the mesolimbic pathway, causing positive symptoms; it is low in the mesocortical pathway to the dorsolateral prefrontal cortex (DLPFC), causing cognitive and negative symptoms; it is low in the mesocortical pathway to ventromedial prefrontal cortex (VMPFC), causing affective and negative symptoms; and it is normal in the nigrostriatal and tuberoinfundibular pathways (upper panel). With administration of a D2 antagonist, dopamine output is reduced throughout the brain (lower panel). This can reduce the positive symptoms of psychosis, although it may also reduce the experience of pleasure or reward, since these emotions are also mediated by the mesolimbic pathway. Reduction of dopamine output in mesocortical pathways would not improve cognitive, negative, or affective symptoms and might even worsen them. In the nigrostriatal and tuberoinfundibular pathways, reduction of dopamine output could lead to extrapyramidal symptoms (EPS) and prolactin elevation, respectively.

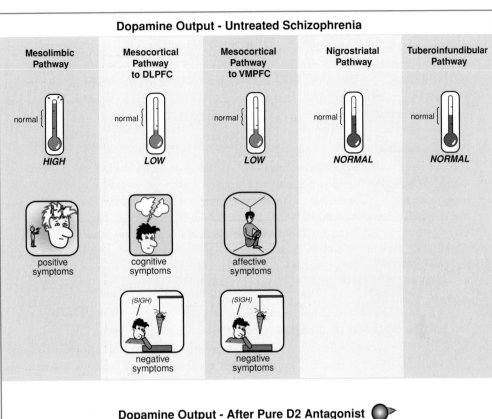

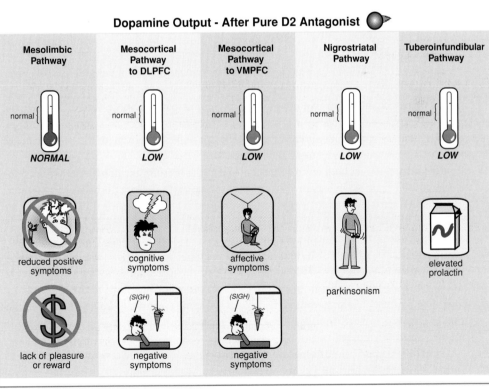

EPS early in treatment may be twice as likely to develop tardive dyskinesia if treatment with a conventional antipsychotic is continued chronically. Also, specific genotypes of dopamine receptors may confer important genetic risk factors for developing tardive dyskinesia with chronic treatment with a conventional antipsychotic. However, risk of a new onset of tardive dyskinesia can diminish considerably after 15 years of treatment with a conventional antipsychotic, presumably because patients who have not developed tardive dyskinesia over this treatment period have lower genetic risk factors.

Prolactin elevation

D2 receptors in the tuberoinfundibular DA pathway are also blocked by conventional antipsychotics, which causes plasma prolactin concentrations to rise, a condition called hyperprolactinemia (Figure 2-6). This is associated with a condition called galactorrhea (i.e., breast secretions) and amenorrhea (i.e., irregular menstrual periods). Hyperprolactinemia may thus interfere with fertility, especially in women. It might also lead to more rapid demineralization of bones, especially in postmenopausal women who are not receiving estrogen replacement therapy. Other possible problems associated with elevated prolactin levels may include sexual dysfunction and weight gain, although the role of prolactin in causing such problems is not clear.

The dilemma of blocking D2 dopamine receptors in all dopamine pathways

It should now be obvious that the use of conventional antipsychotic drugs presents a powerful dilemma. That is, there is no doubt that conventional antipsychotic medications have dramatic therapeutic effects on positive symptoms of psychosis by blocking hyperactive dopamine neurons in the mesolimbic dopamine pathway. However, there are **several** dopamine pathways in the brain. It appears that blocking dopamine receptors in **only one** of them is useful, whereas blocking dopamine receptors in the remaining pathways may be harmful (Figure 2-7).

Specifically, delusions and hallucinations are reduced when mesolimbic D2 receptors are blocked, but this may come at the expense of loss of reward in this same pathway (Figure 2-7). The near shutdown of the mesolimbic dopamine pathway necessary to improve the positive symptoms of psychosis in some patients may contribute to anhedonia, apathy, and negative symptoms of schizophrenia; this may be a partial explanation for the high incidence of smoking and drug abuse among such patients.

In addition to blocking reward mechanisms in the mesolimbic dopamine system, conventional antipsychotic actions in other dopamine systems may cause the negative, cognitive, and affective symptoms of psychosis to be worsened when mesocortical D2 receptors are blocked; EPS and tardive dyskinesia may be produced when nigrostriatal D2 receptors are blocked; and hyperprolactinemia and its complications may be produced when tuberoinfundibular D2 receptors are blocked. The pharmacological quandary here is what to do if one wishes simultaneously to **decrease** dopamine in the mesolimbic dopamine pathway in order to treat positive psychotic symptoms and yet **increase** dopamine in the mesocortical dopamine pathway to treat negative and cognitive symptoms while leaving dopaminergic tone unchanged in both the nigrostriatal and tuberoinfundibular dopamine pathways in order to avoid side effects.

This dilemma may have been solved in part by the atypical antipsychotic drugs described in the following sections and is one of the reasons why the atypical antipsychotics have largely replaced conventional antipsychotic agents in the treatment of schizophrenia and other psychotic disorders throughout the world.

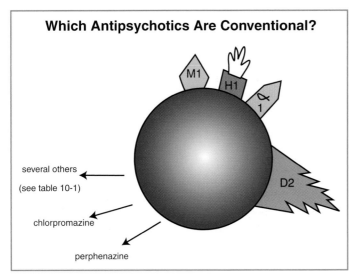

Which Antipsychotics Are Conventional?

M1
H1
α1
several others
(see table 10-1)
chlorpromazine
perphenazine
D2

FIGURE 2-8 Conventional antipsychotic. Shown here is an icon representing a conventional antipsychotic drug. Conventional antipsychotics have pharmacological properties in addition to dopamine D2 antagonism. The receptor profiles differ for each agent, contributing to divergent side-effect profiles. However, some important characteristics that multiple agents share are the ability to block muscarinic cholinergic receptors, histamine-1 receptors, and/or alpha-1 adrenergic receptors.

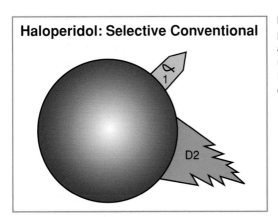

Haloperidol: Selective Conventional

α1
D2

FIGURE 2-9 Haloperidol. Haloperidol pharmacological icon. Haloperidol is a conventional antipsychotic that, in addition to blocking D2 receptors, also inhibits alpha-1 adrenergic receptors. Haloperidol has little or no affinity for muscarinic cholinergic or histaminergic receptors.

Muscarinic cholinergic blocking properties of conventional antipsychotics

In addition to blocking D2 receptors in all dopamine pathways (Figure 2-7), conventional antipsychotics have other important pharmacological properties (Figures 2-8 through 2-13). One particularly important pharmacological action of some conventional antipsychotics is their ability to block muscarinic cholinergic receptors (Figures 2-8, 2-10, and 2-11). This can cause undesirable side effects such as dry mouth, blurred vision, constipation, and cognitive blunting (Figure 2-10). Differing degrees of muscarinic cholinergic blockade may also explain why some conventional antipsychotics have a greater propensity to produce extrapyramidal side effects (EPS) than others. That is, those conventional antipsychotics that cause more EPS are the agents that have only **weak** anticholinergic properties, whereas those conventional antipsychotics that cause fewer EPS are the agents that have **stronger** anticholinergic properties.

How does muscarinic cholinergic receptor blockade reduce the EPS caused by dopamine D2 receptor blockade in the nigrostriatal pathway? This effect seems to be

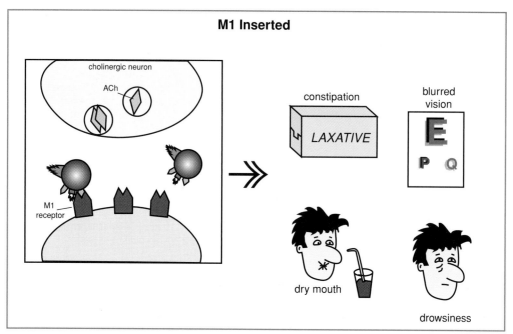

M1 Inserted

cholinergic neuron

ACh

M1 receptor

constipation

LAXATIVE

blurred vision

E
P   Q

dry mouth

drowsiness

FIGURE 2-10 Side effects of muscarinic cholinergic receptor blockade. In this diagram, the icon of a conventional antipsychotic drug is shown with its M1-anticholinergic/antimuscarinic portion inserted into acetylcholine receptors, causing the side effects of constipation, blurred vision, dry mouth, and drowsiness.

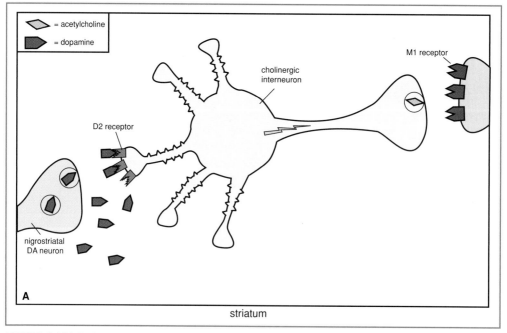

= acetylcholine

= dopamine

M1 receptor

cholinergic interneuron

D2 receptor

nigrostriatal DA neuron

A

striatum

FIGURE 2-11A Reciprocal relationship of dopamine and acetylcholine. Dopamine and acetylcholine have a reciprocal relationship in the nigrostriatal dopamine pathway. Dopamine neurons here make postsynaptic connections with the dendrite of a cholinergic neuron. Normally, dopamine suppresses acetylcholine activity (no acetylcholine being released from the cholinergic axon on the right).

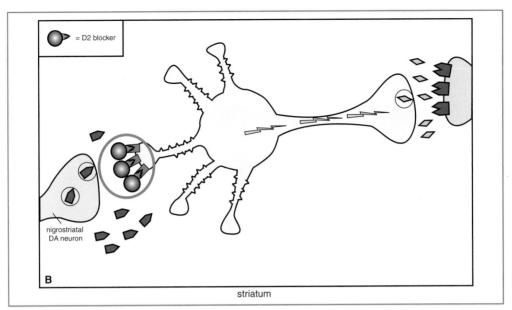

FIGURE 2-11B Dopamine, acetylcholine, and D2 antagonism. This figure shows what happens to acetylcholine activity when dopamine receptors are blocked. As dopamine normally suppresses acetylcholine activity, removal of dopamine inhibition causes an increase in acetylcholine activity. Thus if dopamine receptors are blocked at the D2 receptors on the cholinergic dendrite on the left, then acetylcholine becomes overly active, with enhanced release of acetylcholine from the cholinergic axon on the right. This is associated with the production of extrapyramidal symptoms (EPS). The pharmacological mechanism of EPS therefore seems to be a relative dopamine deficiency and a relative acetylcholine excess.

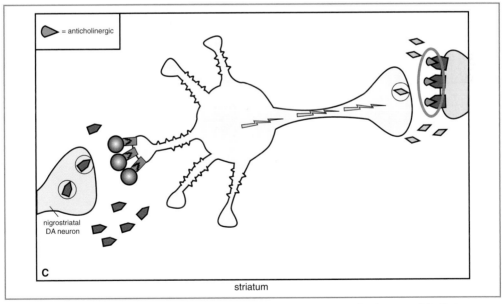

FIGURE 2-11C D2 antagonism and anticholinergic agents. One compensation for the overactivity that occurs when dopamine receptors are blocked is to block the acetylcholine receptors with an anticholinergic agent (M1 receptors being blocked by an anticholinergic on the far right). Thus, anticholinergics overcome excess acetylcholine activity caused by removal of dopamine inhibition when dopamine receptors are blocked by conventional antipsychotics. This also means that extrapyramidal symptoms (EPS) are reduced.

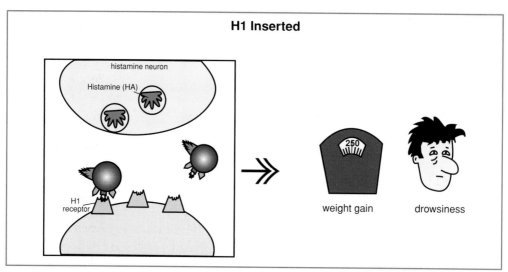

FIGURE 2-12 Histamine 1 receptor antagonism. In this diagram, the icon of a conventional antipsychotic drug is shown with its H1 (antihistamine) portion inserted into histamine receptors, causing the side effects of weight gain and drowsiness.

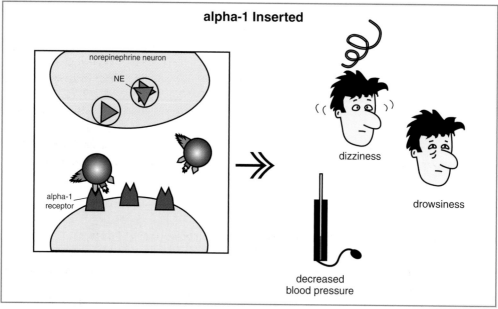

FIGURE 2-13 Alpha-1 receptor antagonism. In this diagram, the icon of a conventional antipsychotic drug is shown with its alpha-1 (alpha-1 antagonist) portion inserted into alpha-1 adrenergic receptors, causing the side effects of dizziness, decreased blood pressure, and drowsiness.

based on the fact that dopamine and acetylcholine have a reciprocal relationship with each other in the nigrostriatal pathway (see Figure 2-11). Dopamine neurons in the nigrostriatal dopamine pathway make postsynaptic connections with cholinergic neurons (Figure 2-11A). Dopamine normally **inhibits** acetylcholine release from postsynaptic nigrostriatal cholinergic neurons, thus suppressing acetylcholine activity there (Figure 2-11A). If dopamine can no longer suppress acetylcholine release because dopamine receptors are being blocked by a conventional antipsychotic drug, then acetylcholine becomes overly active (Figure 2-11B).

One compensation for this overactivity of acetylcholine is to block it with an anticholinergic agent (Figure 2-11C). Thus drugs with anticholinergic actions will diminish the excess acetylcholine activity caused by removal of dopamine inhibition when dopamine receptors are blocked (Figure 2-8 and Figure 2-11C). If anticholinergic properties are present in the same drug with D2-blocking properties, they will tend to mitigate the effects of D2 blockade in the nigrostriatal dopamine pathway. Thus, conventional antipsychotics with potent anticholinergic properties (for example, Figure 2-8) have a lower tendency to cause EPS than conventional antipsychotics with weak anticholinergic properties (Figure 2-9). Furthermore, the effects of D2 blockade in the nigrostriatal system can be mitigated by coadministering an agent with anticholinergic properties. This has led to the common strategy of giving anticholinergic agents along with conventional antipsychotics in order to reduce EPS. Unfortunately, this concomitant use of anticholinergic agents does not lessen the ability of the conventional antipsychotics to cause tardive dyskinesia. It also causes the well-known side effects associated with anticholinergic agents, such as dry mouth, blurred vision, constipation, urinary retention, and cognitive dysfunction (Figure 2-10).

Other pharmacological properties of conventional antipsychotic drugs

Still other pharmacologic actions are associated with the conventional antipsychotic drugs. These include generally undesired blockade of histamine-1 receptors (Figures 2-8 and 2-12), causing weight gain and drowsiness, as well as blockade of alpha-1 adrenergic receptors (Figures 2-8, 2-9, and 2-13), causing cardiovascular side effects such as orthostatic hypotension and drowsiness. Conventional antipsychotic agents differ in terms of their ability to block the various receptors represented in Figures 2-8 and 2-9. [For example, haloperidol, a popular conventional antipsychotic (Figure 2-9), has relatively little anticholinergic or antihistaminic binding activity.] Because of this, conventional antipsychotics differ somewhat in their side-effect profiles even if they do not differ overall in their therapeutic profiles. That is, some conventional antipsychotics are more sedating than others, some have more ability to cause cardiovascular side effects than others, and some have more ability to cause EPS than others.

Risks and benefits of long-term treatment with conventional antipsychotics

Although the conventional antipsychotics reduce positive psychotic symptoms in most patients after several weeks of treatment, discontinuing these drugs causes relapse of psychosis in patients with schizophrenia at the rate of approximately 10 percent per month, so that 50 percent or more have relapsed by 6 months after medication discontinuation. Despite this powerful incentive for patients to continue long-term treatment with conventional antipsychotics to prevent relapse, the unfortunate fact that all dopamine pathways are blocked by these drugs means that many patients do not consider the benefits of long-term treatment worth the resultant problems they cause. This leads many to discontinue treatment, become noncompliant, and relapse with a "revolving door" lifestyle in and out of the hospital. Patients too commonly select the risk of relapse over the subjectively unacceptable side effects of the conventional antipsychotics. Especially unacceptable to patients are motor restlessness and EPS such as akathisia, ridigity, and tremor as well as cognitive blunting and social withdrawal, anhedonia, and apathy. There is even the possibility of a rare but potentially fatal complication called the "neuroleptic malignant syndrome," which is associated with extreme muscular rigidity, high fevers, coma, and even death.

Given these problems with conventional antipsychotics, when are these agents worthwhile to administer? Recently, long-term cardiometabolic risks for some of the atypical antipsychotics have been uncovered (discussed later in this chapter), and this, combined with their higher cost, is leading to a resurgence of interest among some psychopharmacologists in going back to conventional antipsychotic treatment, where the cardiometabolic risks (and costs) may be lower. This may be prudent for some patients who experience a robust therapeutic effect at low doses of a conventional antipsychotic and thus show improvement in positive symptoms without worsening of negative symptoms and without "neurolepsis." Furthermore, if such patients have had 15 years of treatment with a conventional antipsychotic without developing tardive dyskinesia, there may be little additional risk that this will occur with continued treatment with a conventional antipsychotic. It is interesting to note that some so-called first generation conventional antipsychotics (such as loxapine, cyamemazine, and sulpiride) may have the pharmacological properties of an atypical antipsychotic, particularly at low doses (discussed later in this chapter). Administering one of these agents may be a way to treat with a less expensive agent that could potentially have atypical antipsychotic properties.

On the other hand, psychopharmacologists who no longer see tardive dyskinesia in their patients (owing to the conversion of most of their patients to an atypical antipsychotic) must not forget that most patients remain at much higher risk for developing tardive dyskinesia on a conventional antipsychotic than for developing cardiometabolic risks on an atypical antipsychotic, particularly on certain atypical antipsychotics that pose little cardiometabolic risk.

Selecting which antipsychotic to administer to an individual patient thus requires weighing tardive dyskinesia, neurolepsis, EPS, and cardiometabolic risks for that individual against the particular clinical benefits for that same patient in terms of improvement in negative, cognitive, and affective symptoms as well as positive symptoms. In order to make prudent antipsychotic choices for each individual patient, it is necessary to understand the differentiating properties not only of conventional antipsychotics compared to atypical antipsychotics but of each individual antipsychotic drug. These issues are developed in detail throughout this chapter.

What makes an antipsychotic atypical?

What is an "atypical" antipsychotic? From a clinical perspective, it is defined in part by the "atypical" clinical properties that distinguish such drugs from conventional antipsychotics, namely "low EPS" and "good for negative symptoms." From a pharmacological perspective, the atypical antipsychotics as a class may be defined in at least four ways: as "serotonin dopamine antagonists" (Figure 2-14), as "D2 antagonists with rapid dissociation" (Figure 2-39), as "D2 partial agonists (DPA)" (Figure 2-45) or as "serotonin partial agonists (SPA)" at 5HT1A receptors (Figure 2-55). In the following section, we will discuss all four of these proposed pharmacological mechanisms of action of atypical antipsychotics.

Serotonergic neurotransmission and serotonin dopamine antagonism

Here, we will first discuss how some atypical antipsychotics obtain their atypical clinical properties by exploiting the different ways that serotonin and dopamine interact within the key dopamine pathways in the brain. In order to understand the powerful consequences of adding 5HT2A receptor antagonism to D2 antagonism, it is very important to grasp the

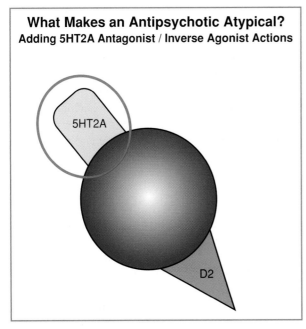

What Makes an Antipsychotic Atypical?
Adding 5HT2A Antagonist / Inverse Agonist Actions

5HT2A

D2

FIGURE 2-14 Serotonin-dopamine antagonist. The "atypicality" of atypical antipsychotics has often been attributed to the coupling of D2 antagonism with serotonin-2A antagonism. Shown here is an icon representing this dual pharmacological action.

principles of serotonin receptor pharmacology and also the nature of serotonin-dopamine interactions in each of the dopamine pathways.

Serotonin synthesis and termination of action

Serotonin is also known as 5-hydroxytryptamine and abbreviated as 5HT. Synthesis of 5HT begins with the amino acid tryptophan, which is transported into the brain from the plasma to serve as the 5HT precursor (Figure 2-15). Two synthetic enzymes then convert tryptophan into serotonin: first tryptophan hydroxylase (TRY-OH) converts tryptophan into 5-hydroxy-tryptophan and then aromatic amino acid decarboxylase (AAADC) converts 5HTP into 5HT (Figure 2-15). After synthesis, 5HT is taken up into synaptic vesicles by a vesicular monoamine transporter (VMAT2) and stored there until it is used during neurotransmission.

The action of 5HT is terminated when it is enzymatically destroyed by MAO and converted into an inactive metabolite (Figure 2-16). Serotonergic neurons themselves contain MAO B, which has low affinity for 5HT; therefore much of 5HT is thought to be enzymatically degraded by MAO A outside of the neuron once 5HT is released. The 5HT neuron also has a presynaptic transport pump for serotonin called the serotonin transporter (SERT), which is unique for 5HT and terminates serotonin's actions by pumping it out of the synapse and back into the presynaptic nerve terminal, where it can be re-stored in synaptic vesicles for subsequent use in another neurotransmission (Figure 2-15).

Serotonin receptors

Serotonin has many different receptor subtypes (Figures 2-17 through 2-20). For a general understanding of 5HT receptors, the reader can begin with the two key receptors that are presynaptic (5HT1A and 5HT1B/D) (Figures 2-17 through 2-19) and several that are postsynaptic (5HT1A, 5HT1B/D as well as 5HT2A, 5HT2C, 5HT3, 5HT4, 5HT5, 5HT6, and 5HT7) (Figure 2-17).

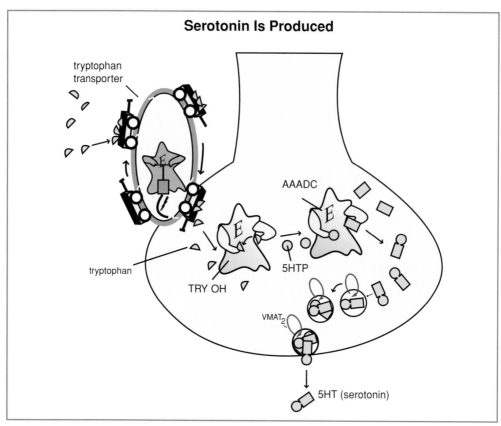

Serotonin Is Produced

tryptophan
transporter

AAADC

tryptophan

5HTP

TRY OH

VMAT$_2$

5HT (serotonin)

FIGURE 2-15 Serotonin is produced. Serotonin (5-hydroxytryptamine [5HT]) is produced from enzymes after the amino acid precursor tryptophan is transported into the serotonin neuron. The tryptophan transport pump is distinct from the serotonin transporter. Once transported into the serotonin neuron, tryptophan is converted by the enzyme tryptophan hydroxylase (TRY-OH) into 5-hydroxytryptophan (5HTP), which is then converted into 5HT by the enzyme aromatic amino acid decarboxylase (AAADC). Serotonin is then taken up into synaptic vesicles via the vesicular monoamine transporter (VMAT2), where it stays until released by a neuronal impulse.

Presynaptic 5HT receptors are autoreceptors and detect the presence of 5HT, causing a shutdown of further 5HT release and 5HT neuronal impulse flow. When 5HT is detected in the synapse by presynaptic 5HT receptors on axon terminals, it occurs via a 5HT1B/D receptor, which is also called a **terminal autoreceptor** (Figure 2-18A). In the case of the 5HT1B/D terminal autoreceptor, 5HT occupancy of this receptor causes a blockade of 5HT release (Figure 2-18B). On the other hand, drugs that block the 5HT1B/D autoreceptor can promote 5HT release. When 5HT is detected in the cell dendrites and cell body, it occurs via a 5HT1A receptor, which is also called a **somatodendritic** autoreceptor (Figure 2-19). This causes a slowing of neuronal impulse flow through the serotonin neuron (Figure 2-19B).

Postsynaptic 5HT receptors translate the chemical signal from serotonin into a signal within the postsynaptic neuron (Figures 2-17 and 2-20). All of these receptors in one way or another regulate various neuronal circuits. More specifically, postsynaptic 5HT1A receptors inhibit cortical pyramidal neurons and are thought to regulate hormones, cognition, anxiety, and depression (Figure 2-20). 5HT2A receptors, on the other hand, excite cortical pyramidal neurons, enhance glutamate release, and inhibit dopamine release while

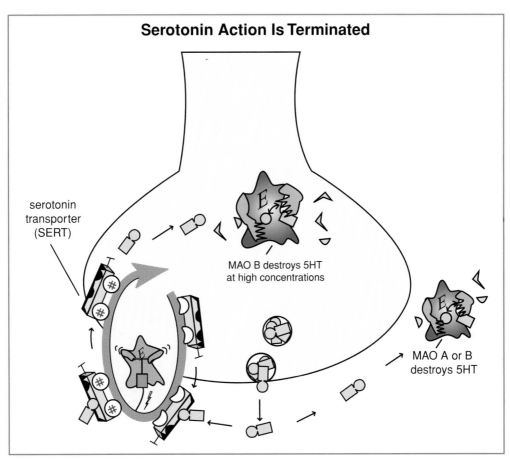

Serotonin Action Is Terminated

serotonin
transporter
(SERT)

MAO B destroys 5HT
at high concentrations

MAO A or B
destroys 5HT

FIGURE 2-16 Serotonin's action is terminated. Serotonin's (5HT) action is terminated by the enzymes monoamine oxidase A (MAO-A) and MAO-B outside the neuron, and by MAO-B within the neuron when it is present in high concentrations. These enzymes convert serotonin into an inactive metabolite. There is also a presynaptic transport pump selective for serotonin, called the serotonin transporter or SERT, that clears serotonin out of the synapse and back into the presynaptic neuron.

playing a role in both sleep and hallucinations (Figure 2-20). 5HT2C receptors regulate both dopamine and norepinephrine release and may play a role in obesity, mood, and cognition (Figure 2-20). 5HT3 receptors regulate inhibitory interneurons in the cortex and mediate vomiting via the vagal nerve (Figure 2-20). 5HT6 receptors are under intense investigation, as they may be key in regulating the release of neurotrophic factors such as brain derived neurotrophic factor (BDNF), which in turn regulates the formation of long-term memory. Finally, the role of 5HT7 receptors is being clarified; these seem to be linked to circadian rhythms, sleep, and mood (Figure 2-20).

5HT1A and 5HT2A receptors have opposite actions in regulating dopamine release

Some serotonin receptors have a major influence on dopamine release; when serotonin acts on them, they can determine whether dopamine release is stimulated or inhibited. Specifically, 5HT1A receptors act as an accelerator for dopamine release, whereas 5HT2A receptors act as a brake on dopamine release (Figure 2-21). How does this happen?

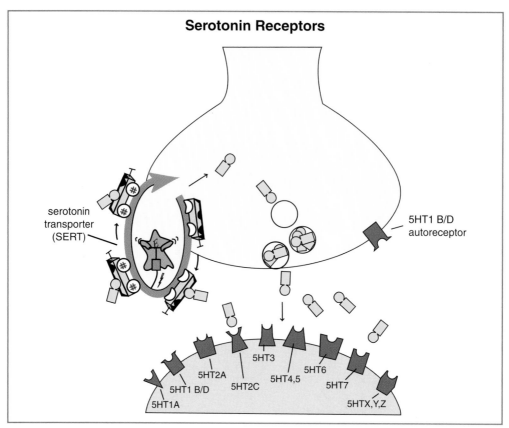

FIGURE 2-17 Serotonin receptors. Receptor subtyping for the serotonergic neuron has proceeded at a very rapid pace. On the presynaptic side, in addition to the well-known serotonin (5HT) transporter, there is a key presynaptic 5HT receptor (5HT1B/D) that functions as an autoreceptor. Several postsynaptic 5HT receptors (5HT1A, 5HT1B/D, 5HT2A, 5HT2C, 5HT3, 5HT4, 5HT6, 5HT7, and many others denoted by 5HTX,Y,Z) are shown here as well.

The 5HT2A receptor is a dopamine brake

Serotonin neurons innervate dopamine neurons either directly via postsynaptic 5HT2A receptors on the dopamine neuron, or indirectly via 5HT2A receptors on GABA interneurons (Figure 2-21). When serotonin is released onto these postsynaptic 5HT2A receptors, the dopamine neuron is inhibited, providing a braking action on dopamine release (lower left of Figure 2-21).

The 5HT1A receptor is a dopamine accelerator

How does serotonin also act as an accelerator to stimulate dopamine release via 5HT1A receptors? Recall that 5HT1A receptors in the somatodendritic region of serotonin neurons are autoreceptors that act to inhibit serotonin release (Figure 2-19). When 5HT1A receptors inhibit serotonin release (Figure 2-19B), the 5HT2A postsynaptic receptors on dopamine neurons cannot be activated (lower right of Figure 2-21). In other words, the 5HT2A dopamine brake is not applied and dopamine neurons will lose the inhibitory action of serotonin via 5HT2A receptors. This lack of 5HT2A inhibition is also known as "disinhibition," which is just a fancy way of saying "turned on." Technically speaking,

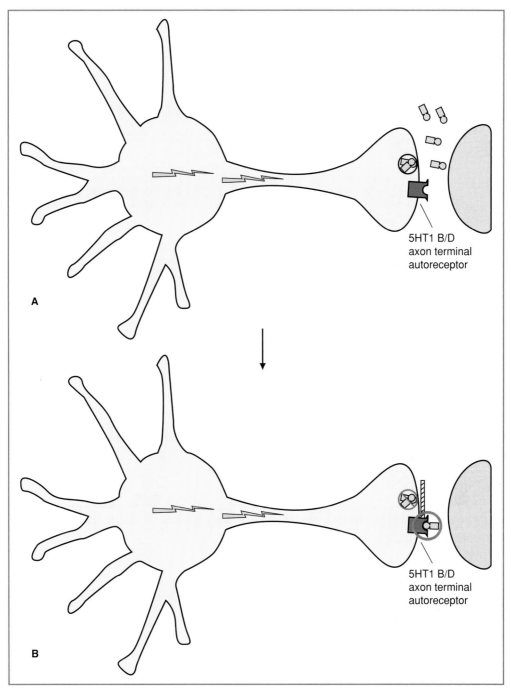

FIGURE 2-18A and B 5HT1B/D autoreceptors. Presynaptic 5HT1B/D receptors are autoreceptors located on the presynaptic axon terminal. They act by detecting the presence of serotonin (5HT) in the synapse and causing a shutdown of further 5HT release. When 5HT builds up in the synapse (**A**), it is available to bind to the autoreceptor, which then inhibits serotonin release (**B**).

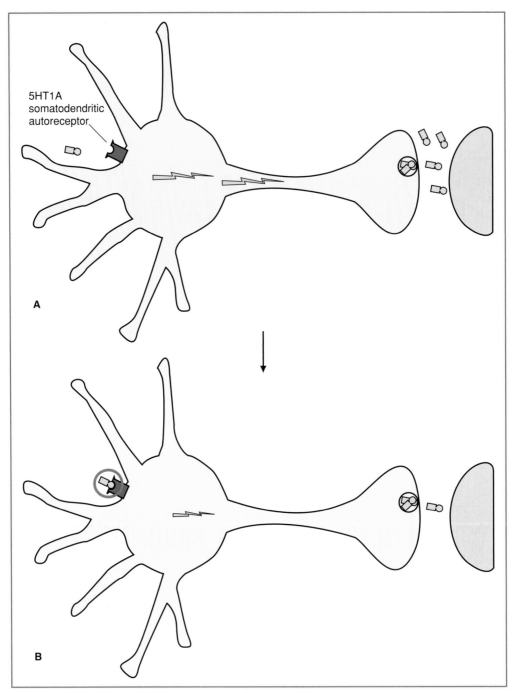

FIGURE 2-19A and B 5HT1A autoreceptors. Presynaptic 5HT1A receptors are autoreceptors located on the cell body and dendrites, and are therefore called somatodendritic autoreceptors (**A**). When serotonin (5HT) binds to these 5HT1A receptors, it causes a shutdown of 5HT neuronal impulse flow, depicted here as decreased electrical activity and a reduction in the release of 5HT from the synapse on the right (**B**).

Possible Functions of Postsynaptic Serotonin Receptors

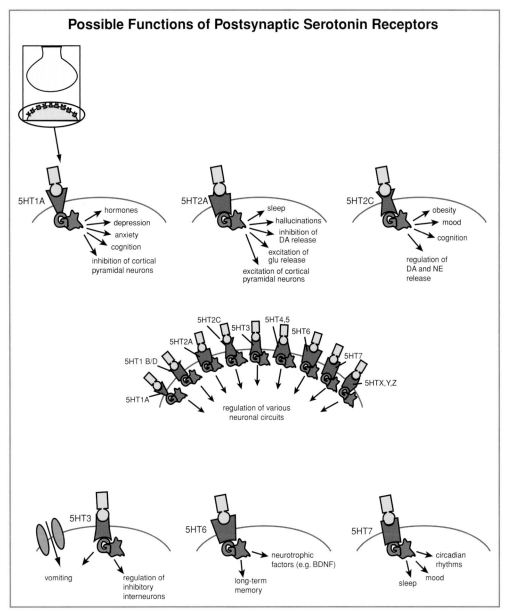

FIGURE 2-20 **Possible functions of postsynaptic serotonin receptors.** Postsynaptic serotonin (5HT) receptors are G protein–linked receptors. 5HT binding to these receptors causes signal transduction and downstream events that regulate various neuronal circuits. In particular, postsynaptic 5HT1A receptors inhibit cortical pyramidal neurons, regulate hormones, and play a role in depression, anxiety, and cognition. 5HT2A receptors excite cortical pyramidal neurons, increase glutamate release, decrease dopamine release, and are involved in sleep and hallucinations. 5HT2C receptors regulate dopamine and norepinephrine release and play a role in obesity, mood and cognition. 5HT3 receptors regulate inhibitory interneurons in the brain and also mediate vomiting via the vagal nerve. 5HT6 receptors may regulate release of neurotrophic factors (e.g., brain-derived neurotrophic factor, or BDNF), which could affect long-term memory. 5HT7 receptors may be involved in circadian rhythms, mood, and sleep.

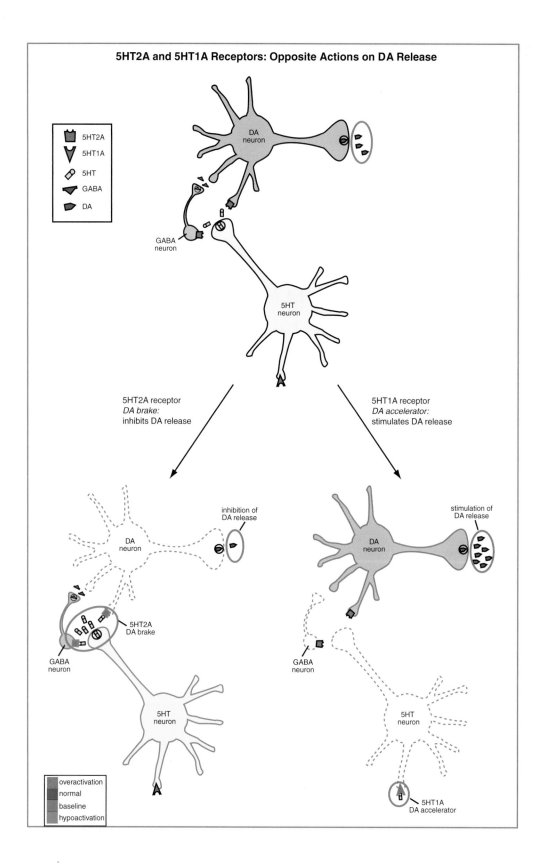

5HT2A and 5HT1A Receptors: Opposite Actions on DA Release

5HT2A receptor
DA brake:
inhibits DA release

5HT1A receptor
DA accelerator:
stimulates DA release

inhibition of
DA release

stimulation of
DA release

activation of 5HT1A autoreceptors disinhibits the dopamine neuron, and thus dopamine release is enhanced (Figure 2-21, lower right). Thus, the presynaptic somatodendritic 5HT1A autoreceptor is a DA accelerator.

5HT2A antagonism makes an antipsychotic atypical
5HT2A antagonists stimulate dopamine release

Many atypical antipsychotics are antagonists at the 5HT2A receptor as well as at the D2 receptor (Figure 2-14). Some research suggests that this antagonist action is actually more precisely described as inverse agonist action at 5HT2A receptors, but the clinical differences between antagonists and inverse agonists are not yet clear. Here we will continue to refer to the actions of atypical antipsychotics at 5HT2A receptors as antagonist actions.

What is so important about 5HT2A antagonist actions of atypical antipsychotics? 5HT2A antagonism can cause dopamine release in certain brain areas (Figure 2-22), and this pharmacological action hypothetically explains the atypical clinical properties of these agents that distinguish them from conventional antipsychotics, namely "low EPS" and "good for negative symptoms." Thus, the 5HT2A receptor "brake" on dopamine release shown in Figure 2-21 and on the left in Figure 2-22 is disrupted by a 5HT2A antagonist, essentially cutting the brake cable, disinhibiting the dopamine neuron, and stimulating dopamine release (Figure 2-22, the right).

5HT2A antagonism reduces EPS

So far, we have shown how serotonin neurons act on the somatodendritic regions of dopamine neurons (Figures 2-21 and 2-22). However, serotonin neurons may also act on the axon terminals of dopamine neurons (Figures 2-23 through 2-26). For example, serotonin actions on nigrostriatal dopamine neurons may occur both at the level of the brainstem in the substantia nigra, where the somatodendritic regions of these dopamine neurons are located, and also in the striatum, where the axon terminals of these dopamine neurons are located (Figure 2-23). In both cases, a 5HT2A receptor mediates the action of serotonin at the dopamine neuron, via either a direct connection between the serotonin neuron and the dopamine neuron or an indirect connection with a GABA interneuron (Figure 2-24A). Specifically, Figure 2-24B shows actions of 5HT2A receptors in the somatodendritic region of the dopamine neuron in the substantia nigra, inhibiting dopamine release in the striatum, as in Figure 2-21, lower left. In addition, the actions of 5HT2A receptors on dopamine axon terminals in the striatum are shown in Figure 2-24C, also inhibiting the release of dopamine in the striatum. A closeup depiction of these actions of 5HT at axon terminal 5HT2A receptors in the striatum is shown in Figure 2-25, where striatal dopamine release

FIGURE 2-21 5HT2A and 5HT1A receptors: opposite actions on DA release. Serotonin (5HT) 1A and 2A receptors influence dopamine (DA) release, either directly or via gamma aminobutyric acid (GABA) neurons. However, these receptors actually have opposite effects on DA release. Specifically, 5HT2A receptors act as a DA brake. When 5HT binds to 5HT2A receptors on postsynaptic DA neurons, this inhibits DA release (bottom left). Similarly, 5HT binding to 5HT2A receptors on GABA interneurons causes GABA release, which in turn inhibits DA release (also bottom left). 5HT1A somatodendritic autoreceptors, on the other hand, act as DA accelerators. That is, when 5HT binds to these receptors, it inhibits 5HT release; thus, 5HT is unable to inhibit DA release, and dopamine release is thus disinhibited, and therefore increased (bottom right).

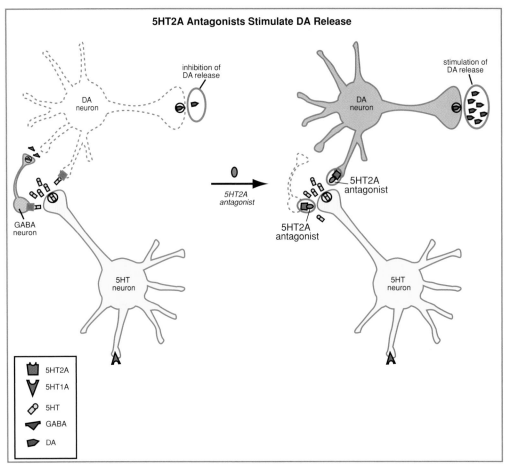

FIGURE 2-22 5HT2A antagonists stimulate DA release. Serotonin (5HT) inhibits dopamine (DA) release via stimulation of 5HT2A receptors (left); when this action is blocked by a 5HT2A antagonist, this leads to an increase in DA release, either by blocking 5HT2A receptors on postsynaptic DA neurons or by blocking 5HT2A receptors on gamma aminobutyric acid (GABA) interneurons (on the right).

(Figure 2-25A) is inhibited by serotonin actions at postsynaptic 5HT2A receptors located at an axoaxonic synapse of a serotonin neuron on a striatal dopamine nerve terminal (Figure 2-25B).

How does 5HT2A antagonist action reduce EPS? The answer to this is shown in Figure 2-26, where both the D2 and 5HT2A antagonist actions of an atypical antipsychotic are illustrated in the striatum. First, the D2 actions of an atypical antipsychotic are shown in Figure 2-26A. In this case, most of the D2 receptors in the striatum are occupied, and if this persisted, it would cause EPS, as this would be no different than the actions of a conventional antipsychotic with pure D2 antagonist actions (Figure 2-1). However, in Figure 2-26B, the additional action of the 5HT2A antagonist is shown. Adding this second action results in disinhibition of the dopamine neuron, which causes stimulation of dopamine release, just as has already been explained and illustrated in Figure 2-22. The result of this increased dopamine release is that dopamine competes with drug at D2 receptors and reduces binding there enough to eliminate EPS (Figure 2-26B).

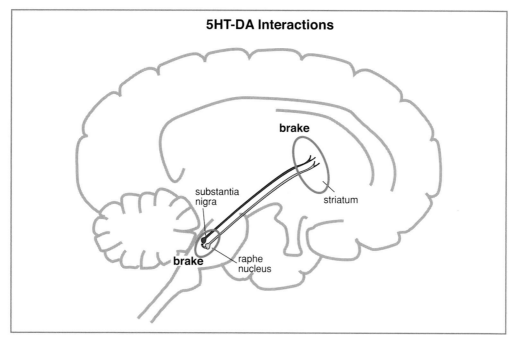

FIGURE 2-23 5HT-DA interactions. Serotonin-dopamine interactions in the nigrostriatal dopamine pathway. Serotonin inhibits dopamine release, both at the level of the dopamine cell bodies in the brainstem substantia nigra and at the level of the axon terminals in the basal ganglia-neostriatum. In both cases, the release of serotonin acts as a brake on dopamine release.

These actions of an atypical antipsychotic with both D2 antagonist actions and 5HT2A antagonist actions are confirmed when imaging D2 receptors in the striatum of patients receiving antipsychotic drugs (Figure 2-27). In the case of a conventional antipsychotic given at clinically effective doses, it is estimated that up to 90 percent of D2 receptors are blocked in every dopamine pathway in the brain. This degree of blockade of D2 receptors in the nucleus accumbens of the mesolimbic dopamine pathway is presumably necessary to reduce positive symptoms of psychosis, but this degree of simultaneous blockade of D2 receptors in the striatum causes EPS and eventually, tardive dyskinesia. An artist's conception of occupancy of 90 percent of D2 receptors by a conventional antipsychotic drug is shown in Figure 2-27A. Real neuroimaging scans with positron emission tomography (PET) ligands are much more complicated, but we know that if we could selectively label the D2 receptors in the striatum after a clinically effective dose of a conventional antipsychotic, a high proportion of D2 receptors in the striatum would be occupied (Figure 2-27A).

However, in the case of an atypical antipsychotic, the number of D2 receptors that are occupied in the striatum is notably less at clinically effective doses (Figure 2-27B). How can this be? Presumably it is due to the actions of drug blocking 5HT2A receptors and leading to increased striatal dopamine release (as shown in Figure 2-26B), which in turn causes dopamine to knock enough drug off D2 receptors that the occupancy drops below the threshold for producing EPS (i.e., presumably less than 70 to 80 percent of D2 receptor occupancy).

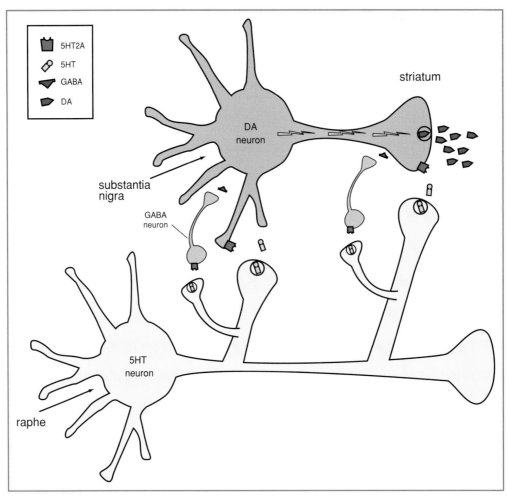

FIGURE 2-24A Serotonin regulation of dopamine release from nigrostriatal dopamine neurons, part 1. Here, dopamine is being freely released from its axon terminal in the striatum because there is no serotonin causing direct or indirect inhibition of dopamine release.

5HT2A antagonism reduces negative symptoms

There is a debate as to how robustly atypical antipsychotics compared to conventional antipsychotics reduce negative symptoms. Some experts believe that atypical antipsychotics do not really reduce negative symptoms but that conventional antipsychotics increase them, presumably due to the induction of secondary negative symptoms related to EPS. If conventional antipsychotics cause EPS and thus secondary negative symptoms but atypical antipsychotics do not (as explained in the section above and illustrated in Figures 2-26 and 2-27), this could explain some of the apparent differences in the severity of negative symptoms in patients taking conventional antipsychotics versus atypical antipsychotics.

However, the lack of production of secondary negative symptoms does not appear to be an adequate explanation for all the reduction in severity of negative symptoms by atypical antipsychotics compared to conventional antipsychotics. Another mechanism that could explain this apparent reduction is that atypical antipsychotics, working through their 5HT2A antagonist properties, may increase dopamine release in hypoactive mesolimbic

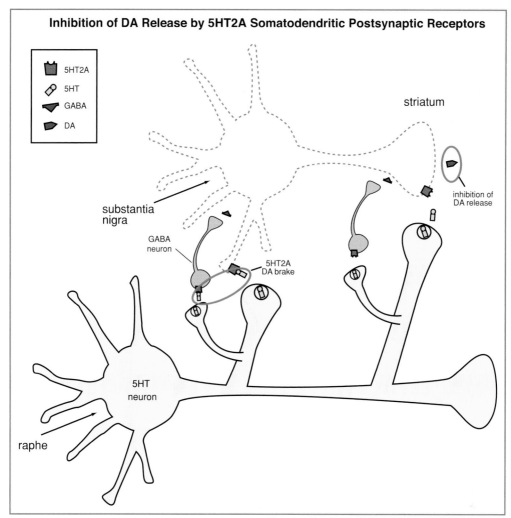

FIGURE 2-24B Serotonin regulation of dopamine release from nigrostriatal dopamine neurons, part 2. Now, serotonin is being released from a synaptic connection projecting from the raphe to the substantia nigra and terminating on somatodendritic postsynaptic serotonin 2A (5HT2A) receptors on dopamine and gamma aminobutyric acid (GABA) neurons (bottom red circle). Because of this, dopamine release from its axonal terminal is now inhibited (top red circle).

pleasure centers. If this were the case to any great extent, one might expect to see an activation of positive symptoms by atypical antipsychotics as well, but this is not observed. Apparently, dopamine release by 5HT2A receptor antagonism in the nucleus accumbens is not as robust as in other brain areas.

What, then, is the mechanism whereby atypical antipsychotics improve the negative, cognitive, and affective symptoms of schizophrenia in those patients in whom these actions are observed? The answer is illustrated in Figure 2-28 where the 5HT2A antagonist actions of atypical antipsychotics are shown to be increasing DA release in prefrontal cortex. Note that no blockade of D2 receptors in the prefrontal cortex is shown, since D2 receptors are not very dense in this part of the brain. Note also that dopamine deficiency can be primary, due to hypoactive mesocortical dopamine neurons (Figure 2-28A), or secondary,

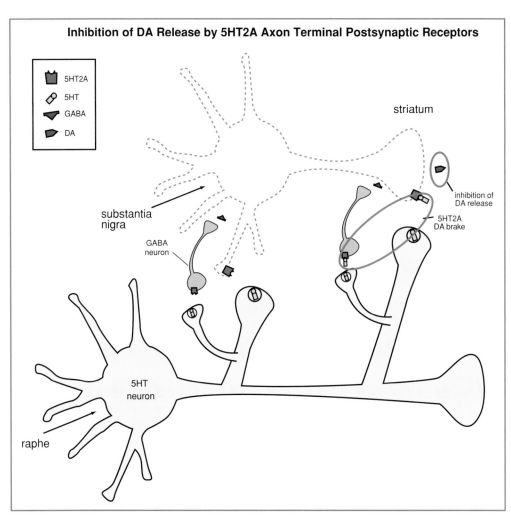

Inhibition of DA Release by 5HT2A Axon Terminal Postsynaptic Receptors

FIGURE 2-24C Serotonin regulation of dopamine release from nigrostriatal dopamine neurons, part 3. Here, serotonin is being released from a synaptic connection projecting from axoaxonal contacts or by volume neurotransmission between serotonergic axon terminals and dopamine axon terminals, resulting in serotonin occupying postsynaptic serotonin 2A (5HT2A) receptors on dopamine and gamma aminobutyric acid (GABA) neurons (bottom red circle). Because of this, dopamine release from its axonal terminal is inhibited (top red circle).

due to high levels of serotonin acting at 5HT2A receptors, causing inhibition of dopamine release (Figure 2-28B). Secondary dopamine deficiency in mesocortical dopamine pathways is sometimes seen in patients taking serotonin selective reuptake inhibitors (SSRIs), which boost the action of serotonin at 5HT2A receptors on mesocortical dopamine neurons, thus producing the side effect of cognitive dulling and affective flattening. Figure 2-28C shows what happens when a 5HT2A antagonist occupies 5HT2A receptors on mesolimbic dopamine neurons: namely, dopamine release is increased. Thus, affective, cognitive, and negative symptoms in schizophrenia may be reduced (Figure 2-28C).

These actions of atypical antipsychotics are confirmed when 5HT2A receptors in the cortex of a patient receiving antipsychotic drugs are imaged (Figure 2-29). In the case of a conventional antipsychotic given at clinically effective doses, essentially no 5HT2A

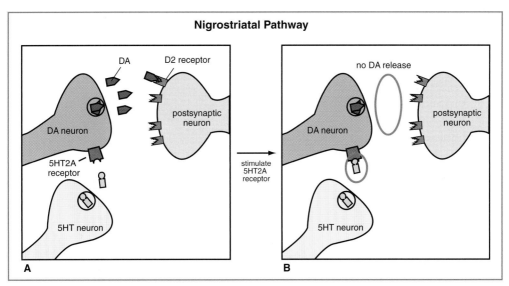

FIGURE 2-25A and B Enlarged view of serotonin (5HT) and dopamine (DA) interactions in the nigrostriatal DA pathway at axon terminals in the striatum. Normally, 5HT inhibits DA release. **(A)** DA is being released because no 5HT is stopping it. Specifically, no 5HT is present at its 5HT2A receptor on the nigrostriatal DA neuron. **(B)** Now DA release is being inhibited by 5HT in the nigrostriatal dopamine pathway. When 5HT occupies its 5HT2A receptor on the DA neuron (lower red circle), this inhibits DA release, so there is no DA in the synapse (upper red circle).

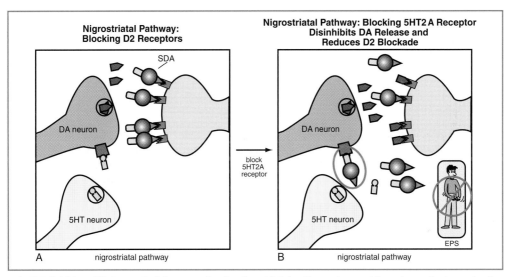

FIGURE 2-26A and B Serotonin 2A antagonists in nigrostriatal pathway. In panel **A** postsynaptic dopamine 2 (D2) receptors are being blocked by a serotonin-dopamine antagonist (SDA) in the nigrostriatal dopamine pathway. This shows what would happen if only the D2 blocking action of an atypical antipsychotic were active – namely, the drug would only bind to postsynaptic D2 receptors and block them. In contrast, panel **B** shows the dual action of the SDAs, in which both D2 and serotonin 2A (5HT2A) receptors are blocked. The interesting thing is that the second action of 5HT2A antagonism actually reverses the first action of D2 antagonism. This happens because dopamine is released when serotonin can no longer inhibit its release. Another term for this is disinhibition. Thus, blocking a 5HT2A receptor disinhibits the dopamine neuron, causing dopamine to pour out of it. The consequence of this is that dopamine can then compete with the SDA for the D2 receptor and reverse the inhibition there. As D2 blockade is thereby reversed, SDAs cause little or no extrapyramidal symptoms (EPS) or tardive dyskinesia.

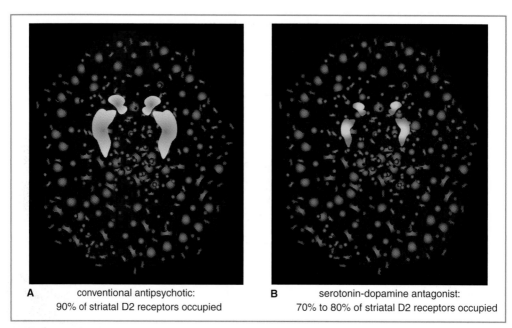

| A | conventional antipsychotic: | B | serotonin-dopamine antagonist: |
| | 90% of striatal D2 receptors occupied | | 70% to 80% of striatal D2 receptors occupied |

FIGURE 2-27A and B Artist's conception of a conventional antipsychotic drug vs. an atypical antipsychotic drug binding to postsynaptic D2 receptors in the nigrostriatal pathway. (A) Autoradiographic and radioreceptor labeling studies in experimental animals as well as positron emission tomography (PET) scans in schizophrenic patients have established that antipsychotic doses of conventional antipsychotic drugs saturate a substantial proportion of the binding capacity of these receptors. Here, bright colors indicate binding to D2 receptors and show that about 90 percent of D2 receptors are being blocked at an antipsychotic dose of a conventional antipsychotic in a schizophrenic patient, which explains why such doses also cause extrapyramidal symptoms (EPS). **(B)** Although this patient is receiving an antipsychotic dose of an atypical antipsychotic, the binding of drug to D2 receptors in the striatum is less intense in color than the scan in panel A, indicating only about 70 to 80 percent blockade of receptors. This reduction is sufficient to put the patient below the threshold for EPS. Thus, this patient has the benefit of the drug's antipsychotic actions without having EPS. Presumably blockade of D2 receptors in the mesolimbic dopamine pathway (not shown), which is the target for reducing positive symptoms of psychosis, is matched for patients in both panels, which is why they both have relief of psychosis.

receptors are occupied in the cortex because conventional antipsychotic drugs do not have high affinity for 5HT2A receptors (Figure 2-29A). However, at clinically effective doses of an atypical antipsychotic, a very high proportion of 5HT2A receptors are occupied (Figure 2-29B). Areas where a 5HT2A antagonist is binding to 5HT2A receptors on mesolimbic dopamine neurons represent areas where dopamine release is presumably enhanced as well. The increased availability of dopamine to areas with hypoactive dopamine release in schizophrenia may lead to improvement in the negative, cognitive, and affective symptoms thought to be mediated by these areas of the brain.

Theoretically, the ideal treatment of schizophrenia would be a drug with actions at clinical doses that fully saturate 5HT2A receptors in the prefrontal cortex (Figure 2-29B) while blocking enough D2 receptors in the mesolimbic area to reduce positive symptoms but not abolish reward; also, the drug would block too few D2 receptors in the nigrostriatal pathway to cause EPS (Figure 2-27B). The atypical antipsychotics with 5HT2A antagonist properties at least as potent as their D2 antagonist properties seem to fulfill that role (see Figures 2-27B and 2-29B).

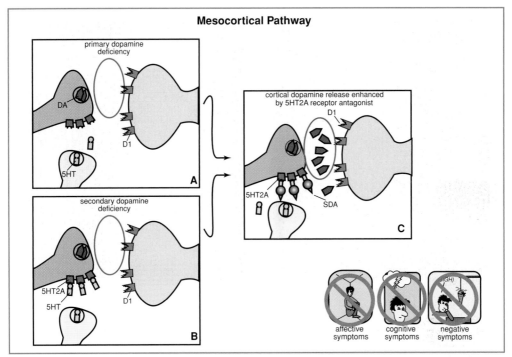

FIGURE 2-28A, B and C Mesocortical pathway and serotonin-dopamine antagonism. The mesocortical dopamine (DA) pathway may mediate affective, cognitive, and negative symptoms in schizophrenia because of a relative deficiency in DA, due either to a primary deficiency (**A**) or to various secondary causes, such as serotonin (5HT) excess (**B**). In either case, blockade of 5HT2A receptors with an atypical antipsychotic should lead to DA release (**C**), which could compensate for the DA deficiency and improve affective, cognitive, and negative symptoms.

5HT2A antagonism may improve positive symptoms

We have already discussed how 5HT1A receptors and 5HT2A receptors regulate dopamine release (Figure 2-21). These same receptors also regulate glutamate release, with 5HT1A receptors acting as brakes to inhibit glutamate release and 5HT2A receptors acting as accelerators to stimulate glutamate release (Figure 2-30). This is the opposite of their regulatory actions on dopamine release (illustrated in Figures 2-21 and 2-22).

The regulatory effects of serotonin on glutamate may play a role in schizophrenia, since it is possible that the stimulatory effects of 5HT2A receptors on glutamate release may be linked to the causation of hallucinations. That is, most hallucinogens are partial agonists at 5HT2A receptors, implicating possible abnormal activation of 5HT2A receptors on cortical glutamate neurons not only in hallucinogen abuse but also in schizophrenia.

Furthermore, in schizophrenia, the action of 5HT2A receptors in enhancing cortical glutamate output (Figure 2-30) can be linked to the pathophysiology of positive symptoms such as hallucinations within a three-neuron circuit: one utilizing serotonin, one utilizing dopamine, and one utilizing glutamate (Figure 2-31). That is, glutamate input via projections to mesolimbic dopaminergic neurons in the VTA can be direct (as shown in Figure 2-31) or indirect (the predominant circuit already shown in Figure 1-39). The direct excitatory input of glutamate descending to the VTA shown in Figure 2-31 is hypothetically

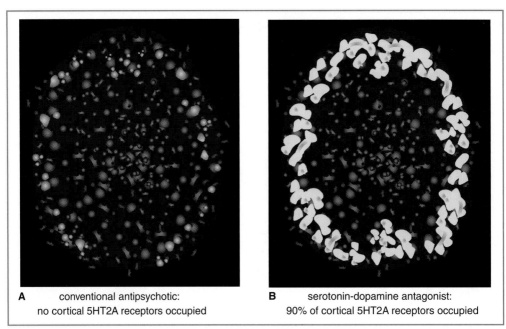

A	conventional antipsychotic:	B	serotonin-dopamine antagonist:
	no cortical 5HT2A receptors occupied		90% of cortical 5HT2A receptors occupied

FIGURE 2-29A and B Artist's conception of a conventional antipsychotic drug vs. an atypical antipsychotic drug binding to postsynaptic serotonin 2A (5HT2A) receptors in the cerebral cortex. (A) Autoradiographic and radioreceptor labeling studies in experimental animals as well as positron emission tomography (PET) scans in schizophrenic patients have established that antipsychotic doses of conventional antipsychotic drugs essentially bind to none of these receptors. Bright colors indicate binding to 5HT2A receptors, and the lack of any receptors lighting up here confirms the lack of binding to cortical 5HT2A receptors. (B) Autoradiographic and radioreceptor labeling studies in experimental animals as well as PET scans in schizophrenic patients have established that 5HT2A receptors in the cortex are essentially saturated by antipsychotic doses of atypical antipsychotic drugs. Presumably dopamine release occurs at the sites where there is 5HT2A binding, which could lead to improvement in cognitive functioning and negative symptoms by a mechanism not possible for conventional antipsychotic agents.

controlled by serotonin projections ascending to glutamatergic cortical pyramidal neurons (as shown in Figure 2-31).

In schizophrenia, activation of 5HT2A receptors in the prefrontal cortex may contribute to positive symptoms of hallucinations by enhancing the excitation of this descending glutamate neuron, which in turn further excites the mesolimbic dopamine neuron it innervates downstream (Figure 2-31A). The take-away message here is that understanding the pharmacology of this three-neuron circuit shows why 5HT2A antagonist actions could reduce positive symptoms such as hallucinations (Figure 2-31B). That is, when 5HT2A antagonists block the serotonergic excitation of cortical pyramidal cells, their glutamate release is reduced, and this lowers the hyperactive drive on the mesolimbic dopamine pathway downstream, thus reducing hallucinations and other positive symptoms.

This idea suggests that the ideal atypical antipsychotic would have not only 5HT2A antagonist actions but also more potent such actions than D2 antagonist actions in order to optimize antipsychotic therapeutic efficacy and reduce the risk of D2-mediated side effects. In fact, this idea has led to proposals that adding a pure 5HT2A antagonist to either a conventional or atypical antipsychotic drug could result in better control of positive symptoms without producing unwanted side effects. The goal would be to achieve perhaps

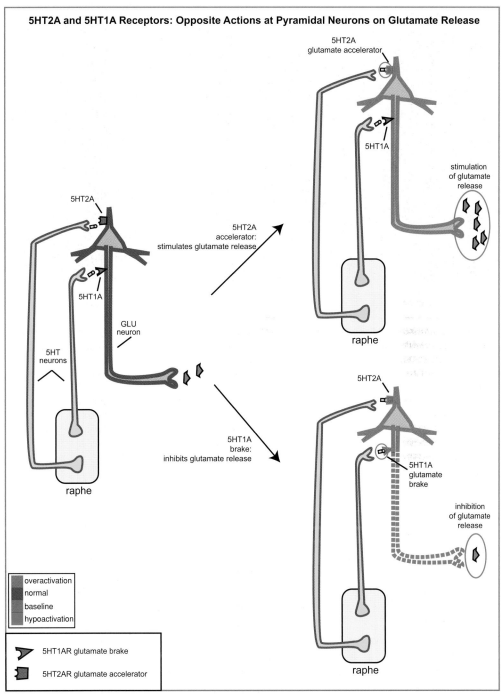

5HT2A and 5HT1A Receptors: Opposite Actions at Pyramidal Neurons on Glutamate Release

FIGURE 2-30 **Effects of 5HT1A and 5HT2A on glutamate release.** Serotonin (5HT) 2A and 5HT1A receptors have opposing actions on glutamate release from cortical pyramidal neurons. Specifically, 5HT2A receptors act as glutamate accelerators, stimulating glutamate release when 5HT binds to them (top right). 5HT1A receptors, on the other hand, act as glutamate brakes. That is, when 5HT binds to cortical 5HT1A receptors, this inhibits glutamate release (bottom right). Thus, the regulatory actions of 5HT2A and 5HT1A on glutamate release are the opposite of their actions on dopamine release, where 5HT2A acts as a brake and 5HT1A acts as an accelerator.

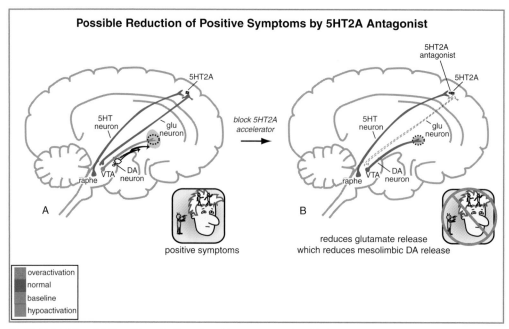

Possible Reduction of Positive Symptoms by 5HT2A Antagonist

FIGURE 2-31A and B Possible reduction of positive symptoms by 5HT2A antagonists. Ascending serotonin (5HT) projections from the raphe to the cortex stimulate release of glutamate from descending glutamatergic cortical pyramidal neurons via postsynaptic 5HT2A receptors. Because descending cortical pyramidal neurons synapse directly with dopaminergic neurons in the ventral tegmental area (VTA), serotonergic actions at 5HT2A receptors can indirectly modulate activity of the mesolimbic dopamine pathway. Thus stimulation of 5HT2A receptors increases glutamate release, which in turn increases dopamine release in the mesolimbic pathway, possibly leading to positive symptoms of psychosis (**A**). On the other hand, blockade of 5HT2A receptors would reduce glutamate release, which in turn would reduce mesolimbic dopamine release (**B**). 5HT2A antagonism is therefore a possible mechanism for reducing positive symptoms of psychosis.

only about 70 to 80 percent blockade of D2 receptors in the mesolimbic dopamine pathway but essentially complete blockade of mesocortical 5HT2A receptors and to do this by "topping up" the antipsychotic with pure 5HT2A antagonism in a second drug. Several selective 5HT2A antagonists and inverse agonists are in testing as add-on treatments to antipsychotics to improve the balance of 5HT2A antagonism to D2 antagonism and thus improve both the efficacy and the tolerability of an antipsychotic. Recently one of these selective 5HT2A agents, actually an inverse agonist at 5HT2A receptors and known as ACP 103, has been reported to enhance the efficacy of risperidone in schizophrenia.

5HT2A antagonist actions reduce hyperprolactinemia

Serotonin and dopamine have reciprocal roles in the regulation of prolactin secretion from the pituitary lactotroph cells. That is, dopamine inhibits prolactin release by stimulating D2 receptors (Figure 2-32), whereas serotonin promotes prolactin release by stimulating 5HT2A receptors (Figure 2-33).

Thus, when D2 receptors are blocked by a conventional antipsychotic, dopamine can no longer inhibit prolactin release, so prolactin levels rise (Figure 2-34). However, in the case of an atypical antipsychotic, there is simultaneous inhibition of 5HT2A receptors, so serotonin can no longer stimulate prolactin release (Figure 2-35). This tends to mitigate the hyperprolactinemia of D2 receptor blockade. Although this is interesting theoretical

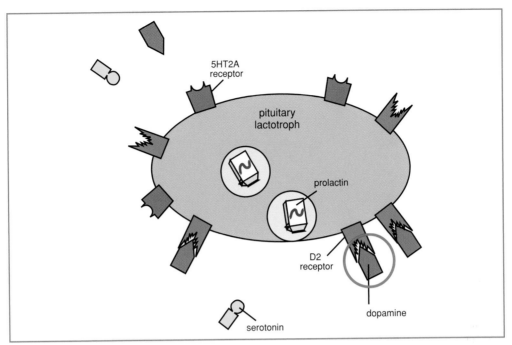

FIGURE 2-32 Dopamine inhibits prolactin. Dopamine inhibits prolactin release from pituitary lactotroph cells in the pituitary gland when it binds to D2 receptors (red circle).

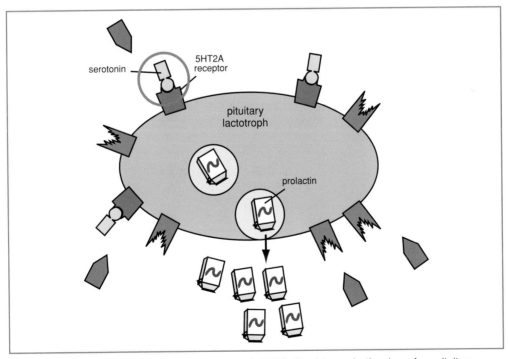

FIGURE 2-33 Serotonin stimulates prolactin. Serotonin (5HT) stimulates prolactin release from pituitary lactotroph cells in the pituitary gland when it binds to 5HT2A receptors (red circle). Thus, serotonin and dopamine have a reciprocal regulatory action on prolactin release.

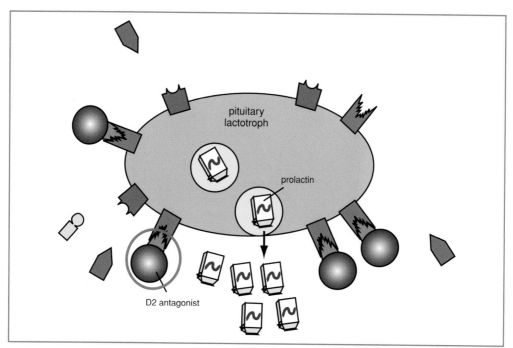

FIGURE 2-34 Conventional antipsychotics and prolactin. Conventional antipsychotic drugs are D2 antagonists and thus oppose dopamine's inhibitory role on prolactin secretion from pituitary lactotrophs. Thus, these drugs increase prolactin levels (red circle).

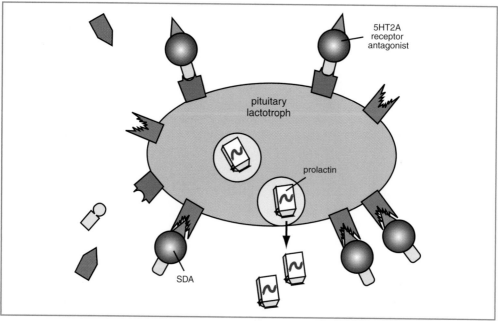

FIGURE 2-35 Atypical antipsychotics and prolactin. This figure shows how serotonin (5HT) 2A antagonism reverses the ability of D2 antagonism to increase prolactin secretion. As dopamine and serotonin have reciprocal regulatory roles in the control of prolactin secretion, one cancels the other. Thus, stimulating 5HT2A receptors reverses the effects of stimulating D2 receptors. The same thing works in reverse, namely, blockade of 5HT2A receptors (shown here) reverses the effects of blocking D2 receptors (shown in Figure 2-34).

pharmacology, in practice, not all serotonin dopamine antagonists reduce prolactin secretion to the same extent and others do not reduce prolactin elevations at all.

"Tuning" dopamine output with serotonin 2A/dopamine 2 antagonists

The actions of antipsychotics can be conceptualized as agents that "tune" dopamine output in malfunctioning neuronal circuits. Schizophrenia is probably not as simple as just "too much" or "too little" dopamine activity in various brain regions. Instead, therapeutic agents must target inefficient information processing in various brain regions by optimizing function. In some cases this may mean increasing dopamine activity, but in others it may mean decreasing dopamine activity. Although a conventional antipsychotic can only decrease dopamine and will do this at D2 receptors throughout the brain (Figure 2-7), antipsychotics with 5HT2A antagonist properties have much more complicated net actions on dopamine activity since they can not only decrease dopamine activity by blocking D2 receptors but also increase dopamine release and thus increase dopamine activity at both D1 and D2 receptors (Figures 2-22 and 2-26 through 2-29).

Which action predominates and in which part of the brain is the subject of intense current investigation, but it is already clear that the addition of 5HT2A antagonist properties to D2 antagonist properties yields a very different type of drug – namely, an atypical antipsychotic agent with therapeutic actions not only on positive symptoms but also on negative, cognitive, and affective symptoms with a significant reduction in the incidence of extrapyramidal side effects and hyperprolactinemia (Figures 2-26 through 2-36).

Clinicians can exploit these properties of atypical antipsychotics by individualizing drug selection and dosage to individual patients, since the exact balance of 5HT2A antagonism versus D2 antagonism differs with different drugs in different parts of the brain, and the ideal balance will be different in individual patients. The trick is to exploit these pharmacological mechanisms to get the best clinical results, often by simultaneous blockade of D2 receptors and 5HT2A receptors with a single drug, which causes nearly the opposite things in different areas of the same brain at the same time! Although there are obviously many other factors at play here and this is an overly simplistic explanation, it is a useful starting point for beginning to appreciate the pharmacological actions of serotonin-2A/dopamine-2 antagonists as a class of atypical antipsychotic drugs.

Numerous therapeutic agents available on the worldwide market have the pharmaco-logical properties of full antagonism of D2 receptors plus antagonism (or inverse agonism) of 5HT2A receptors (Figure 2-37). Each of these will be discussed individually in a later section of this chapter. In addition, several other agents with serotonin-dopamine antag-onism (SDA) pharmacology are in clinical development and may become available in the future (Figure 2-38).

Rapid dissociation from D2 receptors makes an antipsychotic atypical

A second pharmacological mechanism that hypothetically makes an antipsychotic act in an atypical manner is the way in which it binds to D2 postsynaptic receptors: that is, whether it binds "tightly" with long times on the receptor, like a conventional antipsychotic (Figure 2-1), or whether it binds "loosely" and slips off the receptor quickly, with what is termed a rapid "off" time, like some atypical antipsychotics (Figure 2-39). Conventional antipsychotics are known for long-lasting binding to D2 receptors and for this reason are indicated with an icon that has "teeth" in Figures 2-1 and 2-40. Once a conventional antipsychotic binds to the D2 receptor (indicated with grooves for the teeth of the conventional antipsychotic in Figure 2-40), the drug stays for a long time. The consequence of long receptor occupancy

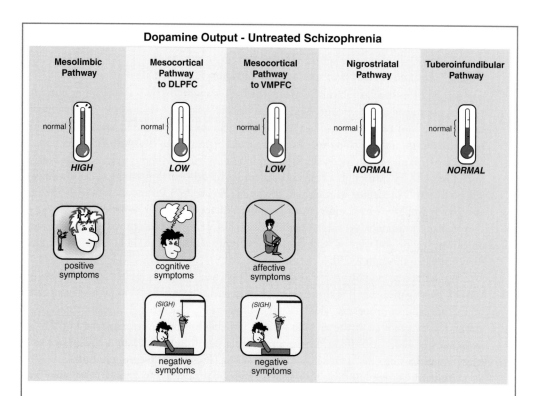

Dopamine Output - Untreated Schizophrenia

Mesolimbic Pathway	Mesocortical Pathway to DLPFC	Mesocortical Pathway to VMPFC	Nigrostriatal Pathway	Tuberoinfundibular Pathway
HIGH	LOW	LOW	NORMAL	NORMAL
positive symptoms	cognitive symptoms	affective symptoms		
	negative symptoms	negative symptoms		

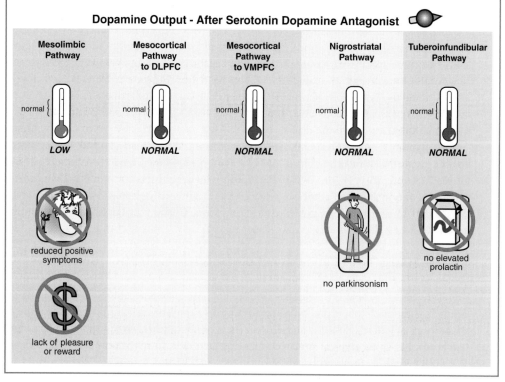

Dopamine Output - After Serotonin Dopamine Antagonist

Mesolimbic Pathway	Mesocortical Pathway to DLPFC	Mesocortical Pathway to VMPFC	Nigrostriatal Pathway	Tuberoinfundibular Pathway
LOW	NORMAL	NORMAL	NORMAL	NORMAL
reduced positive symptoms			no parkinsonism	no elevated prolactin
lack of pleasure or reward				

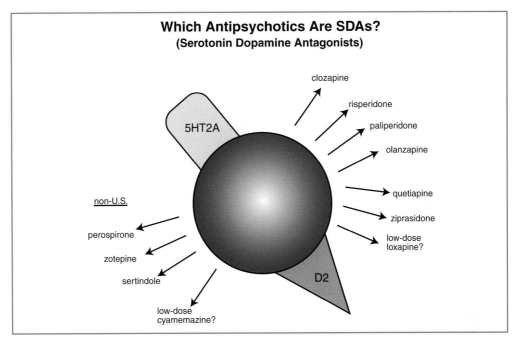

Which Antipsychotics Are SDAs?
(Serotonin Dopamine Antagonists)

FIGURE 2-37 **Serotonin-dopamine antagonists on the market.** Which antipsychotics are SDAs (serotonin 2A/dopamine 2 antagonists)? There are several pharmacological agents available with the dual properties of D2 antagonism and serotonin (5HT) 2A antagonism. These include clozapine, risperidone, paliperidone, olanzapine, quetiapine, and ziprasidone in the United States as well as perospirone, zotepine, and sertindole outside of the United States. In addition, at low doses the conventional antipsychotics loxapine and cyamemazine may be serotonin-dopamine antagonists.

is that conventional antipsychotics outlive their welcome: that is, they don't just stay on the D2 receptor long enough to relieve the positive symptoms of psychosis but instead actually stay too long and thus cause extrapyramidal side effects (Figure 2-41).

By contrast, atypical antipsychotics, even if they also have the 5HT2A antagonist properties discussed above, also have the ability to rapidly dissociate from D2 receptors. This is indicated by a smooth icon for the binding property of an atypical antipsychotic at D2 receptors (Figures 2-14, 2-39, and 2-42). Rapid dissociation from the D2 receptor, or "hit and run" binding, is indicated in Figure 2-42, with the smooth D2 binding surface of the atypical antipsychotic fitting into the D2 receptor (the "hit") but not getting caught in the grooves and thus slipping off (the "run"). Theoretically, such an agent is able to stay at D2 receptors long enough to exert an antipsychotic action but then

FIGURE 2-36 **Integrated theory of schizophrenia and serotonin-dopamine antagonists.** In untreated schizophrenia, dopamine output is high in the mesolimbic pathway, causing positive symptoms; it is low in the mesocortical pathway to dorsolateral prefrontal cortex (DLPFC), causing cognitive and negative symptoms; it is low in the mesocortical pathway to ventromedial prefrontal cortex (VMPFC), causing affective and negative symptoms; and it is normal in the nigrostriatal and tuberoinfundibular pathways (top panel). With administration of a D2/serotonin 2A antagonist, dopamine output is decreased in the mesolimbic pathway, which can reduce the positive symptoms of psychosis, although it may also reduce the experience of pleasure or reward, since these are mediated by the mesolimbic pathway (bottom panel). Any potential decrease in mesocortical dopamine with D2 antagonism may be offset by serotonin 2A antagonism; in fact, the net effect may actually be that dopamine in the cortex is increased, which could reduce cognitive, negative, or affective symptoms. In the nigrostriatal and tuberoinfundibular pathways, the net effect of serotonin-dopamine antagonism may be that dopamine output is unchanged, thus reducing the risk of extrapyramidal symptoms (EPS) or prolactin elevation (bottom panel).

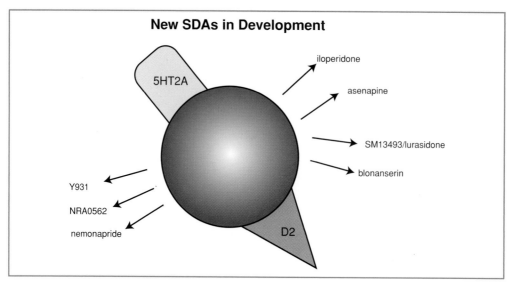

FIGURE 2-38 Serotonin-dopamine antagonists in development. New serotonin-dopamine antagonists currently in development include iloperidone, asenapine, SM13493/lurasidone, blonanserin, nemonapride, NRA0562, and Y931.

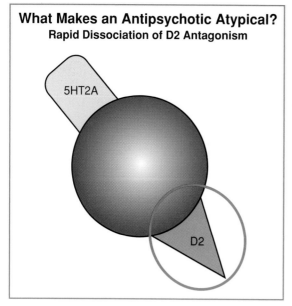

What Makes an Antipsychotic Atypical?
Rapid Dissociation of D2 Antagonism

FIGURE 2-39 Rapid dissociation of D2 antagonism. In addition to serotonin 2A antagonism, the "atypicality" of an antipsychotic may be related to how quickly it dissociates from the D2 receptor, such that long-lasting binding is a feature of conventional antipsychotics and rapid dissociation is a feature of atypical antipsychotics.

leaves prior to producing an extrapyramidal side effect, elevation of prolactin, or worsening of negative symptoms (Figure 2-43). The hit-and-run theory is summarized in Figure 2-44.

One of the interesting clinical aspects of atypical antipsychotics is the observation that they need to be administered less frequently than would be required to keep D2 receptors occupied 24 hours a day. Drugs with short half-lives therefore often need to be administered only once a day. Why is this? It seems possible that continuous receptor occupancy is not

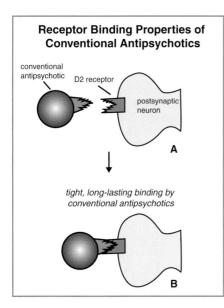

Receptor Binding Properties of Conventional Antipsychotics

conventional antipsychotic

D2 receptor

postsynaptic neuron

A

tight, long-lasting binding by conventional antipsychotics

B

FIGURE 2-40A and B D2 binding of conventional antipsychotics. (**A**) Shown here is an icon for conventional antipsychotic drugs. Because of the biochemical properties of these drugs, their binding to postsynaptic D2 receptors is tight and long-lasting, as shown by the teeth on the binding site of the conventional antipsychotic. The D2 receptor has grooves at which the teeth of the drug can bind tightly. (**B**) Here, the conventional antipsychotic is binding to the postsynaptic D2 receptor, with its teeth locking the drug into the receptor binding site to block it in a long-lasting manner.

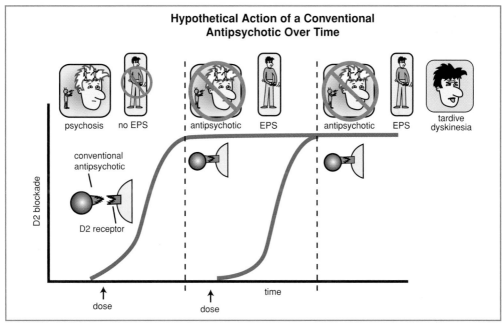

Hypothetical Action of a Conventional Antipsychotic Over Time

psychosis   no EPS   antipsychotic   EPS   antipsychotic   EPS   tardive dyskinesia

D2 blockade

conventional antipsychotic

D2 receptor

time

dose   dose

FIGURE 2-41 Hypothetical action of a conventional antipsychotic over time. This figure shows a curve of D2 receptor blockade after two doses of a conventional antipsychotic as well as the concomitant clinical effects. Prior to dosing a schizophrenic patient with a conventional antipsychotic (far left), there is no D2 receptor blockade, and the schizophrenic patient has positive symptoms of psychosis such as delusions and hallucinations. Also, since there is no drug present, there will be no EPS. Following a dose of a conventional antipsychotic (middle), D2 receptors are blocked so tightly that they both cause antipsychotic actions and induce EPS. Following another dose of a conventional antipsychotic (far right), the D2 receptors stay persistently blocked, so that antipsychotic actions are always associated with EPS and eventually tardive dyskinesia may even occur.

Receptor Binding Properties of Atypical Antipsychotics

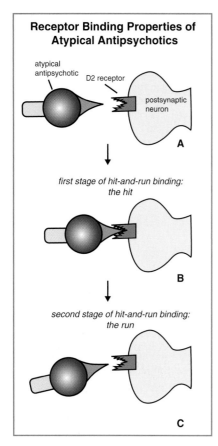

atypical antipsychotic

D2 receptor

postsynaptic neuron

A

first stage of hit-and-run binding: the hit

B

second stage of hit-and-run binding: the run

C

FIGURE 2-42A, B and C Hit-and-run receptor binding properties of atypical antipsychotics. (**A**) Shown here is the icon for atypical antipsychotic drugs. Because of their biochemical nature, the binding of atypical antipsychotics to postsynaptic D2 receptors (shown on the right) is loose, as shown by a smooth binding site for the atypical antipsychotic that does not fit into the teeth of the receptor. (**B**) First stage of hit-and-run binding: the hit. Here the atypical antipsychotic is binding to the D2 receptor. Note that it fits loosely into the D2 receptor without getting locked into the grooves of the receptor as do the conventional antipsychotics. (**C**) Second stage of hit-and-run binding: the run. Since an atypical antipsychotic fits loosely into the D2 receptors, it slips off easily after binding only briefly and then runs away. This is also called rapid dissociation.

required for the desired antipsychotic actions but may in fact contribute to the undesired side effects. Indeed, what may be required for antipsychotic efficacy may be akin to "ringing a bell" by clanging the D2 receptor just once a day. The D2 receptor continues to resonate with antipsychotic actions long after the atypical antipsychotic hits it.

These observations suggest that antipsychotics are atypical because they stay around D2 receptors long enough to cause an antipsychotic action but not long enough to cause side effects. One of the consequences of fast dissociation is that the drug is gone from the receptor until the next dose arrives (Figure 2-43). This means that natural dopamine can bathe the receptor for a while before the next pulse of drug. Perhaps a bit of real dopamine in the nigrostriatal dopamine system is all that is needed to prevent motor side effects. If this happens while there is yet insufficient dopamine in the mesolimbic dopamine system to reactivate psychosis between doses, the drug has atypical antipsychotic clinical properties (Figures 2-42 through 2-44).

The idea of rapid D2 receptor dissociation as a pharmacological property that can explain atypical clinical actions of some antipsychotic drugs is supported by the observation that rapid dissociation from the D2 receptor in vitro is a good predictor of low extrapyramidal side-effect potential in patients. Since rapid dissociation generally also means low potency, this also means that low-potency agents (i.e., those requiring higher milligram doses, such as clozapine and quetiapine) have faster dissociation from the D2 receptor than high-potency agents (i.e., those requiring lower milligram doses, such as risperidone), with

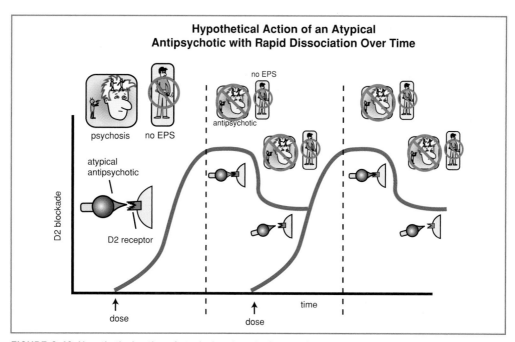

FIGURE 2-43 Hypothetical action of atypical antipsychotic over time. This figure shows a curve of D2 receptor blockade after two doses of an atypical antipsychotic as well as the concomitant clinical effects. Prior to dosing a schizophrenic patient with an atypical antipsychotic (far left), there is no D2 receptor blockade, and the schizophrenic patient has positive symptoms of psychosis, just as in Figure 2-41. Also, since there is no drug present, there will be no extrapyramidal symptoms (EPS). Following a dose of an atypical antipsychotic (middle), D2 receptors are blocked initially, but then the drug slides off the receptor and they are no longer blocked. Theoretically, antipsychotic actions require only initial blockade of D2 receptors, whereas EPS require persistent blockade of D2 receptors. Since the nature of atypical antipsychotic binding is such that the drugs rapidly dissociate from D2 receptors after binding to them, these drugs can have antipsychotic actions without inducing EPS by hitting the D2 receptor hard enough to cause antipsychotic effects and then running before they cause EPS. Since this happens dose after dose (far right), there are persistent and long-lasting antipsychotic actions, but EPS do not develop over time.

intermediate-potency agents such as olanzapine in the middle. This roughly correlates with the abilities of these drugs to cause motor side effects within the group of atypical antipsychotics and also sets them all apart from the conventional antipsychotics. It may also help explain some of the atypical clinical actions of benzamide antipsychotics, such as sulpiride and amisulpride, discussed in the following section, which have low potency at D2 receptors and lack serotonin 2A-antagonist properties yet have some atypical clinical properties.

D2 partial agonism (DPA) makes an antipsychotic atypical

A new class of antipsychotics is emerging that stabilizes dopamine neurotransmission in a state between silent antagonism and full stimulation. This is due to partial agonist actions at the D2 receptor (Figure 2-45). Dopamine partial agonists (DPAs) theoretically bind to the D2 receptor in a manner that is neither too antagonizing, like a conventional antipsychotic ("too cold," with antipsychotic actions but also EPS, as in Figure 2-46A), nor too stimulating, like a stimulant or dopamine itself ("too hot," with positive symptoms of psychosis, as in Figure 2-46B). Instead, a partial agonist binds in an intermediary manner

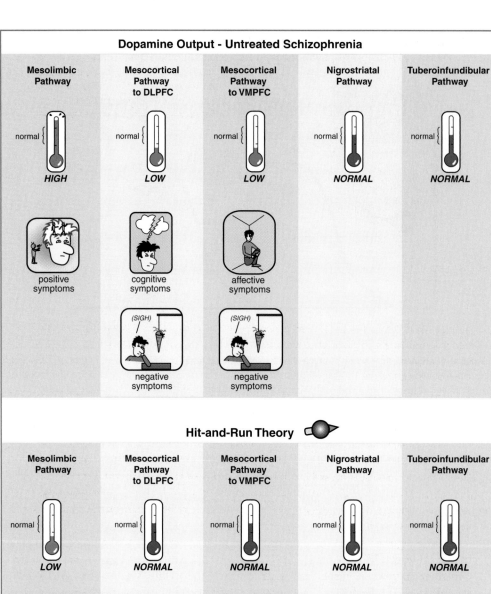

Dopamine Output - Untreated Schizophrenia

Mesolimbic Pathway	Mesocortical Pathway to DLPFC	Mesocortical Pathway to VMPFC	Nigrostriatal Pathway	Tuberoinfundibular Pathway
normal {	normal {	normal {	normal {	normal {
HIGH	**LOW**	**LOW**	**NORMAL**	**NORMAL**
positive symptoms	cognitive symptoms	affective symptoms		
	(SIGH) negative symptoms	(SIGH) negative symptoms		

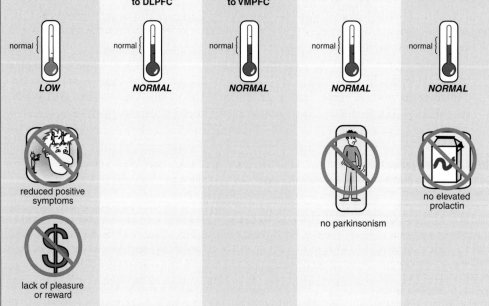

Hit-and-Run Theory

Mesolimbic Pathway	Mesocortical Pathway to DLPFC	Mesocortical Pathway to VMPFC	Nigrostriatal Pathway	Tuberoinfundibular Pathway
normal {	normal {	normal {	normal {	normal {
LOW	**NORMAL**	**NORMAL**	**NORMAL**	**NORMAL**
reduced positive symptoms			no parkinsonism	no elevated prolactin
lack of pleasure or reward				

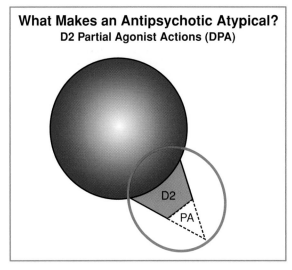

What Makes an Antipsychotic Atypical?
D2 Partial Agonist Actions (DPA)

FIGURE 2-45 D2 partial agonism. What makes an antipsychotic atypical? D2 partial agonist actions (DPA). A third property that may render an antipsychotic atypical is that of partial dopamine 2 antagonism. These agents may stabilize dopamine neurotransmission in a state between silent antagonism and full stimulation.

("just right," with antipsychotic actions but no EPS, as in Figure 2-46C). For this reason, partial agonists that get the balance "just right" between full agonism and complete antagonism are sometimes called "Goldilocks" drugs. However, as we will see, this explanation is an oversimplification.

Partial agonists have the intrinsic ability to bind receptors in a manner that causes signal transduction from the receptor to be intermediate between full output and no output (Figure 2-47). The naturally occurring neurotransmitter generally functions as a full agonist and causes maximum signal transduction from the receptor it occupies (Figure 2-47, top), whereas antagonists essentially shut down all output from the receptor they occupy and make them "silent" in terms of communicating with downstream signal transduction cascades (Figure 2-47, middle). Partial agonists cause receptor output that is more than the silent antagonist but less than the full agonist (Figure 2-47, bottom). Thus many degrees of partial agonism between these two extremes are possible.

Partial agonist actions have unique functional and clinical consequences. Dopamine partial agonists (DPAs) used to treat schizophrenia reduce D2 hyperactivity in mesolimbic dopamine neurons to a degree that is sufficient to exert an antipsychotic action on positive symptoms, even though they do not completely shut down the D2 receptor, as a conventional

---

FIGURE 2-44 Integrated theory of schizophrenia and hit-and-run actions. In untreated schizophrenia, dopamine output is high in the mesolimbic pathway, causing positive symptoms; is low in the mesocortical pathway to dorsolateral prefrontal cortex (DLPFC), causing cognitive and negative symptoms; is low in the mesocortical pathway to ventromedial prefrontal cortex (VMPFC), causing affective and negative symptoms, and is normal in the nigrostriatal and tuberoinfundibular pathways (upper panel). With administration of an agent that rapidly dissociates from D2 receptors, dopamine output is decreased in the mesolimbic pathway, which can reduce the positive symptoms of psychosis, although it may also reduce the experience of pleasure or reward since these are mediated by the mesolimbic pathway (lower panel). Theoretically, decreased dopamine in mesocortical pathways may require persistent blockade of D2 receptors, and thus worsening of affective, cognitive, or negative symptoms may not occur with agents that dissociate rapidly. Similarly, decreased dopamine in the nigrostriatal and tuberoinfundibular pathways may require persistent blockade of D2 receptors; thus, agents that dissociate rapidly may have reduced risk for extrapyramidal symptoms (EPS) and prolactin elevation, respectively (lower panel).

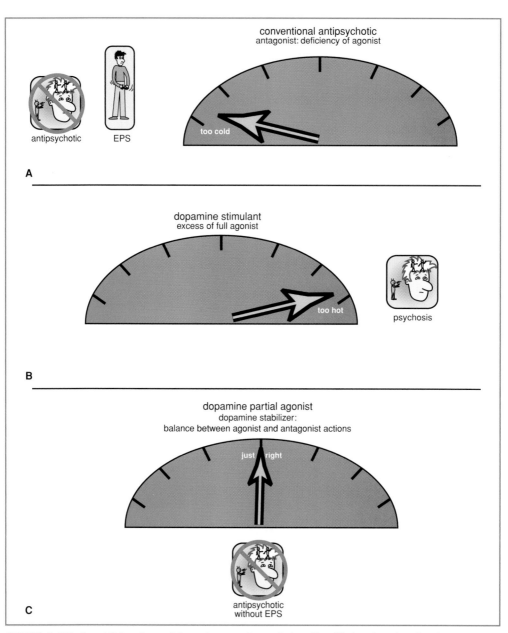

FIGURE 2-46A, B and C Spectrum of dopamine neurotransmission. Simplified explanation of actions on dopamine. (**A**) Conventional antipsychotics bind to the D2 receptor in a manner that is "too cold"; that is, they have powerful antagonist actions while preventing agonist actions and thus can reduce positive symptoms of psychosis but also cause extrapyramidal symptoms (EPS). (**B**) D2 receptor agonists, such as dopamine itself, are "too hot" and can therefore lead to positive symptoms. (**C**) D2 partial agonists bind in an intermediary manner to the D2 receptor and are therefore "just right" with antipsychotic actions but no EPS.

antipsychotic does (Figure 2-48). At the same time, DPAs reduce dopamine activity in the nigrostriatal system to a degree that is insufficient to cause EPS (Figure 2-49). Only a small amount of signal transduction through D2 receptors in the striatum seems to be necessary for a DPA to avoid EPS, and this seems to be the property of DPAs used to

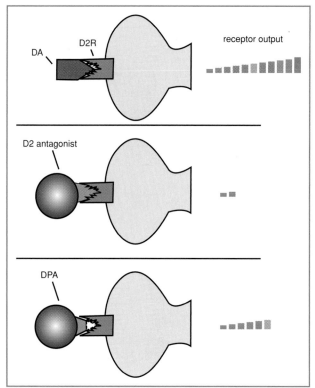

FIGURE 2-47 Dopamine receptor output. Dopamine itself is a full agonist and causes full receptor output (top). Conventional antipsychotics are full antagonists and allow little if any receptor output (middle). The same is true for atypical antipsychotics that are serotonin dopamine antagonists. However, D2 partial agonists can partially activate dopamine receptor output and cause a stabilizing balance between stimulation and blockade of dopamine receptors (bottom).

treat schizophrenia (Figure 2-49). Full agonists, antagonists, and partial agonists may cause different changes in receptor conformation, which lead to a corresponding range of signal transduction output from the receptor (Figure 2-50). The effects of DPAs on dopamine output are summarized in Figure 2-51.

Antipsychotics that act as DPAs include not only aripiprazole but also a new agent called bifeprunox (Figure 2-52). Older agents that may have DPA actions include amisulpride and possibly even low doses of sulpiride, but the partial agonist properties of amisulpride or sulpiride are not well characterized with modern techniques. Many new DPAs are in development (Figure 2-53), and several others have been tested and dropped from further development (Figure 2-54). Bifeprunox is in late stage development in several countries, and related compounds SLV313 and SLV314 are early in clinical testing (Figure 2-53). ACP-104 is a clozapine metabolite that may have DPA actions, but it is still in early testing, and many other compounds shown in Figure 2-53 are also in early testing.

The plethora of new DPAs establishes the point that there is a spectrum of partial agonist action, and clinical testing has shown that too much agonism is not acceptable for a DPA in the treatment of schizophrenia (Figure 2-54). This is perhaps best demonstrated by the successful development of aripiprazole, compared to the failure of a related compound from the same laboratory, OPC 4293. That is, OPC 4293 is a partial agonist that is closer to a full agonist on the DPA spectrum than is aripiprazole (Figure 2-54). This compound did show the ability to improve negative symptoms of schizophrenia, but it caused worsening of positive symptoms, similar to the psychotomimetic actions of a stimulant. Aripiprazole was then developed with a DPA profile closer to the antagonist part of the spectrum and

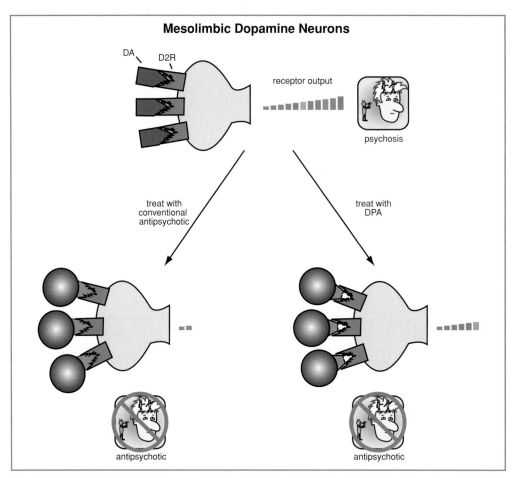

FIGURE 2-48 Dopamine partial agonist in mesolimbic pathway. Excessive dopamine output from mesolimbic dopamine neurons causes psychosis. Both conventional antipsychotics and dopamine partial agonists (DPAs) reduce this output. Although the reduction in dopamine output is not as robust for DPAs (lower right) as it is for the conventional antipsychotics (lower left), dopamine output is reduced sufficiently by a DPA yet with enough stabilization to produce a comparable degree of antipsychotic action to conventional antipsychotics.

has proven to be an atypical antipsychotic without psychotomimetic actions and without significant EPS in most patients.

Several other DPAs that are "too hot" on the spectrum are shown in Figure 2-54. Although there has not been sufficient head-to-head testing of the agents listed as DPAs in Figure 2-52 to determine how they may be distinguishable from each other or exactly where they should be placed along the partial agonist spectrum, hints from both preclinical and clinical investigations suggest that bifeprunox may be closer to the full agonist part of the spectrum than aripiprazole, whereas amisulpride and sulpiride may be closer to the silent antagonist part of the spectrum than aripiprazole. Although it does appear that sulpiride is too close to a silent antagonist to have an ideal clinical profile, it is not clear what the clinical differences are for agents within the effective portion of the DPA spectrum. Perhaps different patients will have better responses to one of these agents versus another, but establishing where different agents may lie on the DPA spectrum and what clinical significance this may have will require much further testing.

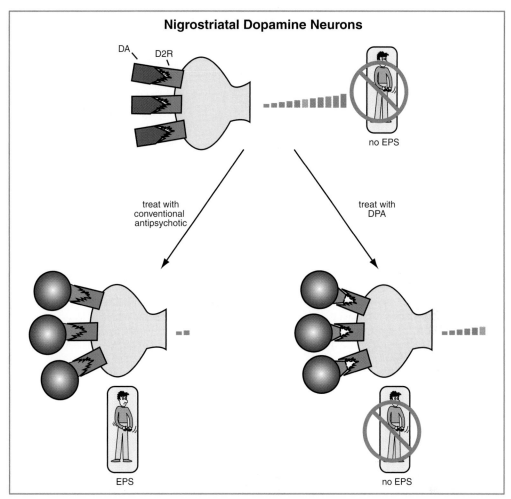

FIGURE 2-49 Dopamine partial agonist and nigrostriatal pathway. Dopaminergic tone in nigrostriatal neurons must be maintained for optimal motor functioning. Conventional antipsychotics reduce this tone so much that extrapyramidal symptoms (EPS) are produced (lower left). On the other hand, dopamine partial agonists allow continuing dopaminergic tone in these neurons, so that EPS are not present (lower right).

5HT1A partial agonist (SPA) actions make an antipsychotic atypical

The fourth pharmacological mechanism that may contribute to the atypical clinical properties of an antipsychotic is the ability of some of these agents to act at 5HT1A receptors either as full agonists or partial agonists (serotonin partial agonist, or SPA) (Figure 2-55). We have already discussed the 5HT2A antagonist actions of some atypical antipsychotics, and have also contrasted the regulatory influence of 5HT1A receptors with 5HT2A receptors on dopamine release (Figure 2-21) and on glutamate release (Figure 2-30). Thus, agonist actions at 5HT1A receptors would be expected to increase dopamine release (Figure 2-21) and reduce glutamate release (Figure 2-30). Enhanced dopamine release by SPA action in the striatum would theoretically improve extrapyramidal actions; enhanced dopamine release by SPA action in the pituitary would theoretically reduce the risk of hyperprolactinemia; and enhanced dopamine release by SPA action in the prefrontal cortex would theoretically improve negative, cognitive, and affective symptoms of schizophrenia.

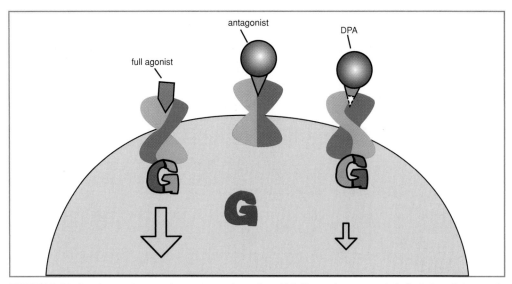

FIGURE 2-50 Agonist spectrum and receptor conformation. This figure shows an artist's depiction of changes in receptor conformation in response to full agonists versus antagonists versus partial agonists. With full agonists, the receptor conformation is such that there is robust signal transduction through the G protein–linked second messenger system of D2 receptors (on the left). Antagonists, on the other hand, bind to the D2 receptor in a manner that produces a receptor conformation that is not capable of any signal transduction (middle). Partial agonists, such as a dopamine partial agonist (DPA), cause a receptor conformation such that there is an intermediate amount of signal transduction (on the right). However, the partial agonist does not induce as much signal transduction (on the right) as a full agonist (on the left).

Reduced glutamate release by SPA action in prefrontal cortex could theoretically reduce positive symptoms. Thus, 5HT1A agonist action has similar net effects to 5HT2A antagonism. Some drugs have both 5HT1A agonist actions and 5HT2A antagonist actions, an action that could be additive or synergistic (Figure 2-56). Other drugs have SPA actions without 5HT2A antagonist actions; furthermore SPA actions can be combined either with D2 antagonism or with DPA to create an atypical antipsychotic drug (Figure 2-56).

Receptor binding properties and pharmacokinetics of antipsychotics

Over two dozen antipsychotic drugs are in clinical use; and so far in this chapter we have discussed pharmacological properties that are shared among some drugs in this class and how those actions are linked to therapeutic efficacy and certain side effects. Many

FIGURE 2-51 Integrated theory of schizophrenia and dopamine partial agonists. In untreated schizophrenia, dopamine output is high in the mesolimbic pathway, causing positive symptoms; it is low in the mesocortical pathway to dorsolateral prefrontal cortex (DLPFC), causing cognitive and negative symptoms; it is low in the mesocortical pathway to ventromedial prefrontal cortex (VMPFC), causing affective and negative symptoms; and it is normal in the nigrostriatal and tuberoinfundibular pathways (upper panel). Dopamine partial agonists decrease dopamine output in comparison to dopamine but allow more dopamine output than a dopamine antagonist (bottom panel). Thus, dopamine output is decreased in the mesolimbic pathway, which can reduce the positive symptoms of psychosis, but the decrease may not be sufficient to affect the experience of pleasure or reward (bottom panel). Because dopamine output in mesocortical pathways is likely already too low, dopamine partial agonists may actually increase dopamine output there and thus potentially improve cognitive, negative, or affective symptoms (bottom panel). In the nigrostriatal and tuberoinfundibular pathways, theoretically, dopamine partial agonism would not reduce dopamine output sufficiently to cause extrapyramidal symptoms (EPS) or prolactin elevation (bottom panel).

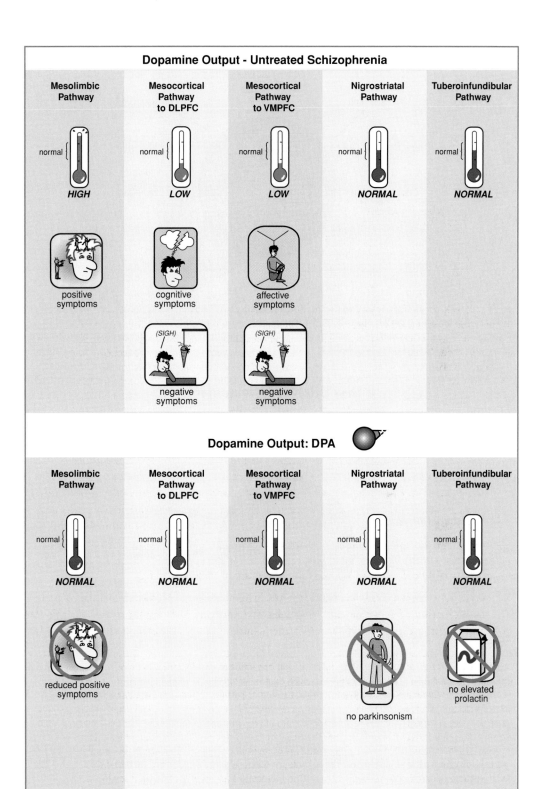

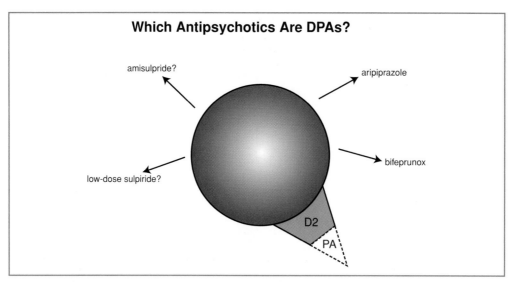

FIGURE 2-52 Dopamine partial agonists on the market. Which antipsychotics are DPAs? Dopamine partial agonists that are currently available or soon to be available include aripiprazole, bifeprunox, possibly amisulpride, and perhaps sulpiride when used at low doses.

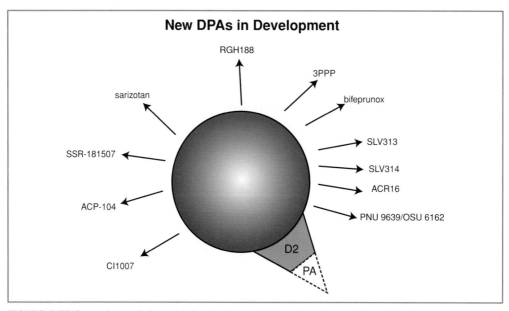

FIGURE 2-53 Dopamine partial agonists in development. New dopamine partial agonists in development include RGH188, 3PPP, bifeprunox, SLV313, SLV314, ACR16, PNU 9639/OSU 6162, CI1007, ACP-104, SSR181507, and sarizotan.

drugs in the antipsychotic class have additional binding properties at receptors other than the dopamine and serotonin receptors discussed above, and many of these drugs also have additional side effects, such as cardiometabolic risk and sedation. In many cases, there is good evidence to link pharmacological actions with clinical actions, but in other cases these links are only hypothetical or even tenuous. In the following section, we will review a number of receptor interactions for antipsychotic drugs and show where there may be

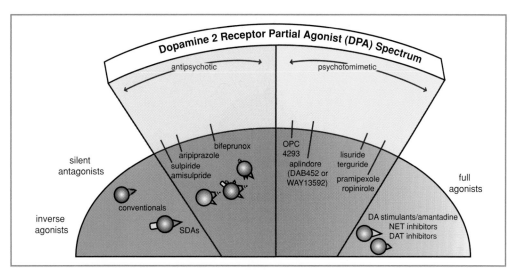

FIGURE 2-54 Spectrum of dopamine partial agonists. Dopamine partial agonists may themselves fall along a spectrum, with some having actions closer to a silent antagonist and others having actions closer to a full agonist. Agents with too much agonism (such as failed agent OPC 4293) may be psychotomimetic and thus not effective antipsychotics. Instead, partial agonists that are closer to the antagonist end of the spectrum (such as aripiprazole or bifeprunox) seem to have favorable profiles. Amisulpride and sulpiride may be very partial agonists, with their partial agonist clinical properties more evident at lower doses.

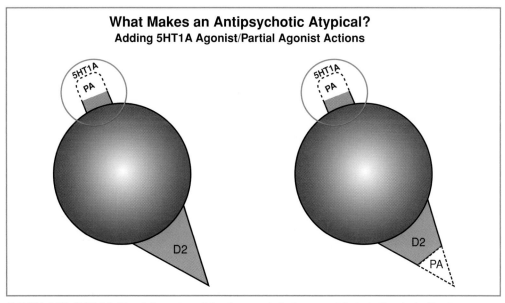

FIGURE 2-55 5HT1A full/partial agonism. A fourth property that may contribute to the atypicality of an antipsychotic is full or partial agonism of serotonin 1A receptors. Agonism of serotonin 1A receptors can increase dopamine release, which could improve affective, cognitive, and negative symptoms while also reducing the risk of extrapyramidal symptoms (EPS) and prolactin elevation. Serotonin 1A agonism can also decrease glutamate release, which could indirectly reduce positive symptoms of psychosis.

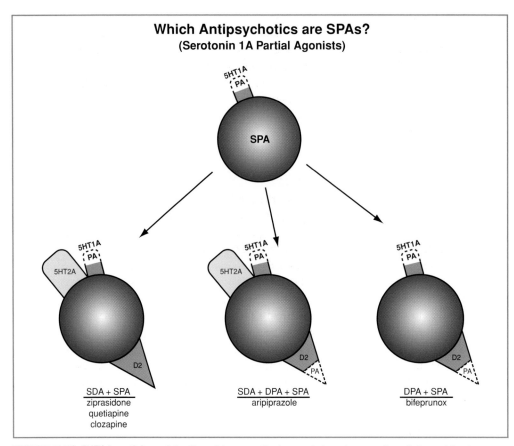

Which Antipsychotics are SPAs?
(Serotonin 1A Partial Agonists)

SPA

SDA + SPA	SDA + DPA + SPA	DPA + SPA
ziprasidone	aripiprazole	bifeprunox
quetiapine		
clozapine		

FIGURE 2-56 5HT1A partial agonists. Ziprasidone, quetiapine, and clozapine are all partial agonists at serotonin (5HT) 1A receptors, in addition to being antagonists at 5HT2A receptors. Aripiprazole is not only a partial agonist at D2 receptors but also an antagonist at 5HT2A receptors and a partial agonist at 5HT1A receptors. Bifeprunox is partial agonist at both D2 and 5HT1A receptors.

potential links between pharmacology and clinical actions. Wherever there is evidence of differentiation among the many members of the antipsychotic class, we will emphasize potential pharmacological explanations for clinical distinctions. Pharmacokinetic properties as well as neurotransmitter receptor binding actions and clinical effects are discussed for antipsychotics in general and for fifteen important antipsychotics in particular.

Links between antipsychotic binding properties and clinical actions

Antipsychotics have perhaps the most complicated pattern of binding to neurotransmitter receptors of any drug class in psychopharmacology. So far, we have concentrated on just three receptors: the D2 dopamine receptor, the 5HT2A receptor, and the 5HT1A receptor. In reality, there are at least a dozen more receptors to which one or another of the antipsychotic drugs also bind (Figure 2-57A). Scientists are just beginning to unravel the clinical significance of these receptor actions, but it is clear that many of them are clinically relevant, contributing to therapeutic actions (Figure 2-57B), side effects (Figure 2-57C), and the clinical differentiation between one agent in this class and another (discussed later in this section and illustrated in Figures 2-90 through 2-104).

Although the actions of these drugs on the various receptors are fairly well established, the link of this receptor binding to clinical actions remains hypothetical, with some links better established than others. We have already discussed the side effects mediated by unwanted D2 receptor blockade, namely extrapyramidal side effects, tardive dyskinesia, hyperprolactinemia, and worsening of negative, cognitive, and affective symptoms in schizophrenia. Here we tackle the possible pharmacological mechanisms involved in mediating two other important side effects: cardiometabolic risk and sedation (Figures 2-57A, 2-58, and 2-66). Later, we will attempt to link other pharmacological properties to both the efficacy and differential side effects of individual atypical antipsychotics (Figures 2-90 through 2-104).

Cardiometabolic risk and antipsychotics

Atypical antipsychotics have been on the market for over a decade, and only now is it becoming clear that some of these agents are associated with significant cardiometabolic risk (Tables 2-2 through 2-4) and with pharmacological actions that may mediate this cardiometabolic risk (Figure 2-58). At first, weight gain and obesity were clearly linked to atypical antipsychotics (Table 2-2 and Figure 2-59), but more recently, increased risk for dyslipidemia, diabetes, accelerated cardiovascular disease, and premature death have been linked to certain drugs in this class as well (Tables 2-3 and 2-4; Figures 2-60 through 2-65).

All of us in western civilization and particularly in the United States, live in a society experiencing an epidemic of obesity and diabetes. The "metabolic highway" begins with increased appetite and weight gain and progresses to obesity, insulin resistance, and dyslipidemia with increases in fasting triglyceride levels (Figure 2-60). Ultimately, hyperinsulinemia advances to pancreatic beta cell failure, prediabetes, and then diabetes. Once diabetes is established, risk for cardiovascular events is further increased, as is the risk of premature death (Figure 2-60).

Cardiovascular disease and diabetes are illnesses determined by both the environment and genetics. Lifestyle factors such as poor diet, lack of exercise, stress, and smoking interact with genetic risk factors such as family history of cardiovascular disease and diabetes associated with genes coding for subtle molecular abnormalities that appear to "bias" the body towards developing cardiovascular disease and diabetes. In the twenty-first century, the schizophrenic patient thus comes to treatment with the same environmental cardiometabolic risk factors that affect all of us. In addition, there is some indication that whatever genes add risk for serious mental illness may also add incremental risk for cardiometabolic disorders. For these reasons, it was not recognized early following the introduction of atypical antipsychotics that some of these agents enhanced cardiometabolic risk beyond these background factors of genes and environment (see Tables 2-2 through 2-4 and Figures 2-58 through 2-65).

As already mentioned, the first indication that certain atypical antipsychotics are associated with increased cardiometabolic risk was the recognition that weight gain, sometimes profound, is associated with some antipsychotics (Table 2-2). Receptors associated with increased weight gain are the H1 histamine receptor and the 5HT2C serotonin receptor; when these receptors are blocked, particularly at the same time, patients can experience weight gain (Table 2-2 and Figures 2-58 and 2-59). Such weight gain is at least in part due to enhanced appetite in hypothalamic eating centers (Figure 2-59), although peripheral factors unrelated to appetite may also be involved in antipsychotic-induced weight gain. Antipsychotics associated with the greatest degree of weight gain are those that have the most potent antagonist actions simultaneously at H1 and 5HT2C receptors (Table 2-2 and Figures 2-58 and 2-59; see also Figures 2-90 through 2-104). Since weight gain

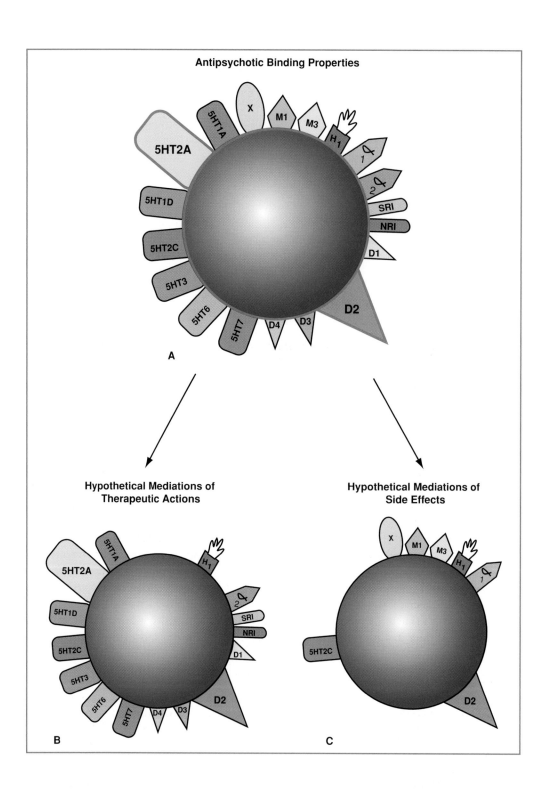

Antipsychotic Binding Properties

A

Hypothetical Mediations of
Therapeutic Actions

B

Hypothetical Mediations of
Side Effects

C

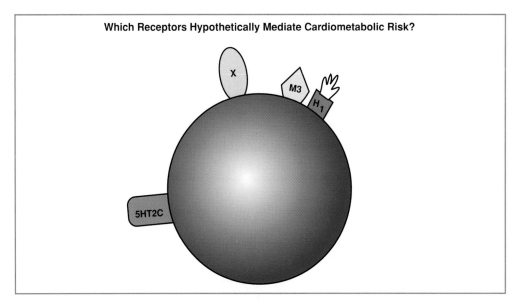

FIGURE 2-58 Receptors mediating cardiometabolic risk. Which receptors hypothetically mediate cardiometabolic risk? Serotonin-2C, muscarinic-3, and histamine-1 receptors as well as receptors yet to be identified (signified here as receptor X), are all hypothetically linked to cardiometabolic risk. In particular, antagonism of serotonin-2C and histamine-1 receptors is associated with weight gain, while antagonism at muscarinic-3 receptors can impair insulin regulation. An unknown receptor X may be involved in the rapid production of insulin resistance and may also rapidly cause elevated fasting plasma triglyceride levels in some patients who experience increased cardiometabolic risk on certain atypical antipsychotics.

can lead to obesity, obesity to diabetes, and diabetes to cardiac disease along the metabolic highway (Figure 2-60), it seemed feasible at first that weight gain might explain all the other cardiometabolic complications linked to treatment with those atypical antipsychotics that cause weight gain (Table 2-2).

However, it now appears that the cardiometabolic risk of certain atypical antipsychotics cannot simply be explained by increased appetite and weight gain, even though they certainly do represent the first steps down the slippery slope toward cardiometabolic complications (Figure 2-61). That is, some atypical antipsychotics can elevate fasting triglyceride levels and cause increased insulin resistance in a manner that cannot be explained by weight gain alone (Tables 2-3 and 2-4; Figures 2-62 and 2-63; see also Figures 2-90 through 2-104). When dyslipidemia and insulin resistance occur, this moves a patient along the

---

FIGURE 2-57A, B and C Pharmacological properties of atypical antipsychotics. Atypical antipsychotics have some of the most complex mixtures of pharmacological properties in psychopharmacology. (**A**) Beyond antagonism of serotonin (5HT) 2A and D2 receptors, agents in this class interact with multiple other receptor subtypes for both dopamine and serotonin, including 5HT1A, 5HT1D, 5HT2C, 5HT3, 5HT6, 5HT7, the 5HT transporter, and D1, D3, and D4. Atypical antipsychotics may have effects on other neurotransmitter systems as well, with inhibition of the norepinephrine transporter as well as muscarinic-1, muscarinic-3, histamine-1, alpha-1 adrenergic, and alpha-2 adrenergic receptors. In addition, some atypical antipsychotics may have actions that alter cellular insulin resistance and increase fasting plasma triglyceride levels, hypothetically due to action at receptors that are not yet well understood, signified by receptor X in this picture. Some of these multiple pharmacological properties can contribute to the therapeutic effects of atypical antipsychotics (**B**), whereas others can contribute to their side effects (**C**). No two atypical antipsychotics have identical binding properties, which probably helps to explain why they all have distinctive clinical properties.

TABLE 2-2 Atypical antipsychotics and risk of weight gain: FDA and experts agree on three tiers of risk

Antipsychotic	Risk for Weight Gain
Clozapine	+++
Olanzapine	+++
Risperidone*	++
Quetiapine	++
Ziprasidone	+/−
Aripiprazole	+/−

*Risperidone's active metabolite paliperidone likely poses the same risk of weight gain as risperidone itself.
FDA, US Food and Drug Administration.

TABLE 2-3 Atypical antipsychotics and cardiometabolic risk: FDA and experts disagree on one versus three tiers of risk

	Cardiometabolic/Dyslipidemia/Diabetes Risk		
Antipsychotic	Expert consensus	CATIE	FDA
Clozapine	Definite risk	ND	Diabetes warning
Olanzapine	Definite risk	Definite risk	Diabetes warning
Risperidone*	Inconclusive	Intermediate	Diabetes warning
Quetiapine	Inconclusive	Definite risk	Diabetes warning
Ziprasidone	+/− limited data	Low-risk	Diabetes warning
Aripiprazole	+/− limited data	ND	Diabetes warning

*Risperidone's active metabolite paliperidone likely poses the same cardiometabolic risk as risperidone itself.
ND, not done (clozapine and aripiprazole not studied in early phases of this trial).
CATIE, Clinical Antipsychotic Trials of Intervention Effectiveness.
FDA, US Food and Drug Administration.

TABLE 2-4 Are there "metabolically friendly" atypical antipsychotics? Low-risk agents for weight gain and cardiometabolic illness

Antipsychotic	Cardiometabolic Risk
Ziprasidone	Low
Aripiprazole	Low
Amisulpride	Possibly low but not well studied
Bifeprunox	Possibly low, studies in progress

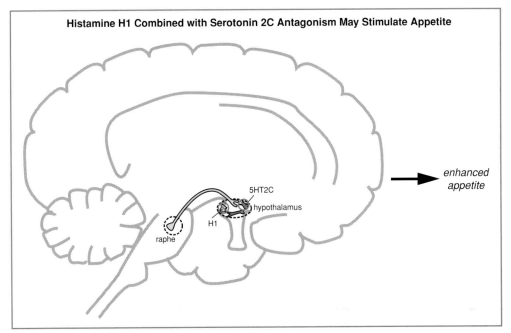

FIGURE 2-59 H1 combined with 5HT2C antagonism. Histamine 1 (H1) combined with serotonin-2C antagonism may stimulate appetite. Antagonism of serotonin-2C and/or H1 receptors can lead to weight gain, perhaps at least in part due to stimulation of appetite regulated by the hypothalamus.

metabolic highway toward diabetes and cardiovascular disease (Figure 2-60). Although this happens in many patients with weight gain alone, it also occurs in some patients who take atypical antipsychotics prior to gaining weight, as though there were an acute receptor-mediated action of these drugs on insulin regulation.

This hypothesized mechanism is indicated as receptor X on the drug icon in Figures 2-57 and 2-58 and on the icons for those agents hypothesized to have this action on insulin resistance and fasting triglycerides (see Tables 2-3 and 2-4 and Figures 2-90 through 2-104). To date, the mechanism of this increased insulin resistance and elevation of fasting triglycerides has been vigorously pursued but has not yet been identified. The rapid elevation of fasting triglycerides on initiation of some antipsychotics and the rapid fall of fasting triglycerides on discontinuation of such drugs (Table 2-3) is highly suggestive that an unknown pharmacological mechanism causes these changes, although this remains speculative. The hypothetical actions of atypical antipsychotics with this postulated receptor action are shown in Figure 2-62, where adipose tissue, liver, and skeletal muscle all develop insulin resistance in response to administration of certain antipsychotic drugs (e.g., high-risk drugs listed in Table 2-3 but not metabolically friendly drugs listed in Table 2-4), at least in certain patients.

Whatever the mechanism of this effect, it is clear that fasting plasma triglycerides and insulin resistance can be elevated significantly in some patients taking certain antipsychotics (Tables 2-3 and 2-4) and that this enhances cardiometabolic risk, moves such patients along the metabolic highway (Figure 2-60), and functions as a second step down the slippery slope toward the diabolical destination of cardiovascular events and premature death (Figure 2-63). This does not happen in all patients taking an antipsychotic (Tables 2-3 and 2-4), but the development of this problem can be detected by monitoring

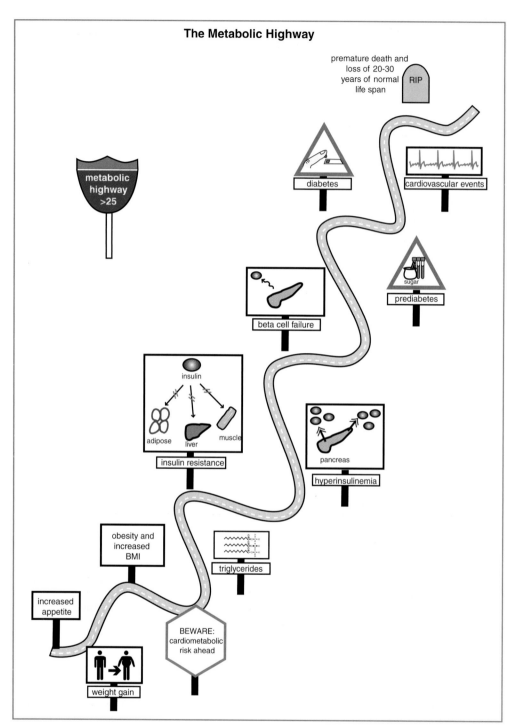

FIGURE 2-60 Metabolic highway. The metabolic highway depicts stages of metabolic changes and illnesses that progressively increase risk of cardiovascular disease and premature death. The "entrance ramp" for the metabolic highway may be increased appetite and weight gain that leads to a body mass index (BMI) greater than 25. This can progress to obesity, insulin resistance, and dyslipidemia, with increases in fasting triglyceride levels. Ultimately, hyperinsulinemia advances to pancreatic beta cell failure, prediabetes, and then diabetes. Diabetes in turn increases risk for cardiovascular events as well as premature death.

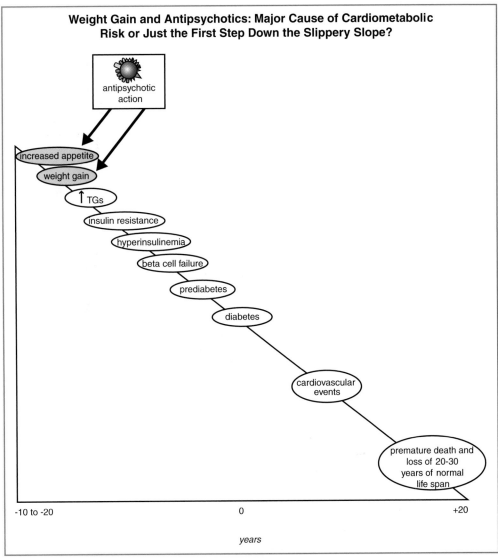

FIGURE 2-61 Weight gain and slippery slope. Weight gain and antipsychotics: major cause of cardiometabolic risk or just the first step down the slippery slope? Rather than being the only risk or even the single major cardiometabolic risk caused by atypical antipsychotics, weight gain associated with increased appetite and that leads ultimately to obesity, appears to be just the first step down the slippery slope of cardiometabolic risk factors leading to premature death. Other cardiometabolic risks caused by atypical antipsychotics are shown in subsequent figures.

(Figures 2-66 through 2-68), and it can be managed easily when it does occur (Figures 2-67 and 2-69).

Another rare but life-threatening cardiometabolic problem is known to be associated with atypical antipsychotics: namely, an association with the sudden occurrence of diabetic ketoacidosis (DKA) or the related condition hyperglycemic hyperosmolar syndrome (HHS) (Figures 2-64 and 2-65). The mechanism of this complication is under intense investigation and is probably complex and multifactorial. In some cases, it may be that patients

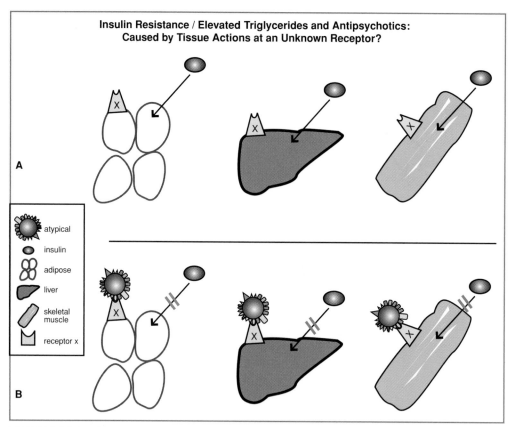

FIGURE 2-62 Insulin resistance, elevated triglycerides, and antipsychotics: caused by tissue actions at an unknown receptor? Some atypical antipsychotics may lead to insulin resistance and elevated triglycerides independently of weight gain, although the mechanism is not yet established. This figure depicts a hypothesized mechanism in which antipsychotic binds to receptor X at adipose tissue, liver, and skeletal muscle to cause insulin resistance.

with undiagnosed insulin resistance, prediabetes, or diabetes who are in a state of compensated hyperinsulinemia on the metabolic highway (Figure 2-60) become decompensated when given an atypical antipsychotic agent because of some pharmacological mechanism associated with these drugs.

One hint for the cause in some patients taking agents such as olanzapine and clozapine is antagonism of the M3 muscarinic cholinergic receptor (Figures 2-57, 2-58, 2-64 and 2-65; see also Figures 2-90 and 2-91). That is, it is known that insulin secretion is regulated in part by parasympathetic cholinergic neurons that innervate the pancreas and act on postsynaptic M3 receptors localized on pancreatic beta cells, the cells that secrete insulin (Figure 2-64A and B). Preclinical research suggests that agents that can block the M3 cholinergic receptor in the pancreatic beta cell may reduce insulin release (Figure 2-64C). If this occurs in a patient dependent on cholinergic regulation of insulin release, it could be a factor in causing insulin deficiency and lead to DKA/HHS. This remains speculative, and many patients have no problem with insulin secretion when M3 receptors are blocked, so this may be just one of several possible mechanisms that could explain the induction of DKA/HHS only in vulnerable patients taking atypical antipsychotics. Because of the risk of DKA/HHS, it is important to know the patient's location along the metabolic

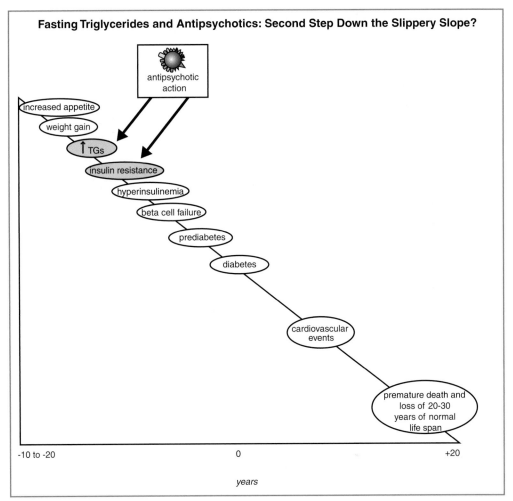

Fasting Triglycerides and Antipsychotics: Second Step Down the Slippery Slope?

antipsychotic action

increased appetite

weight gain

↑ TGs

insulin resistance

hyperinsulinemia

beta cell failure

prediabetes

diabetes

cardiovascular events

premature death and loss of 20-30 years of normal life span

-10 to -20   0   +20

years

FIGURE 2-63 Fasting triglycerides and antipsychotics: second step down the slippery slope?
Antipsychotic-induced elevation of triglycerides (TGs) and insulin resistance may be the second step down the slippery slope of increased cardiometabolic risk. These actions can be independent of weight gain and occur prior to significant weight gain, which suggests that they are mediated by an unknown receptor where certain atypical antipsychotics may interact to cause this risk.

highway (Figure 2-60) prior to prescribing an antipsychotic, particularly if the patient has hyperinsulinemia, prediabetes, or diabetes. It is also important to monitor (Figures 2-66 through 2-68) and manage the metabolic response of the patient to administration of an antipsychotic (Figures 2-67 through 2-69).

There are at least three stops along the metabolic highway where a psychopharmacologist should monitor a patient taking an atypical antipsychotic (Figure 2-66) and manage the cardiometabolic risks of atypical antipsychotics (Tables 2-2, 2-3 and 2-4; Figure 2-67). This starts with monitoring weight and body mass index to detect weight gain and the development of diabetes (Figure 2-66). It also means getting a baseline of fasting triglyceride levels and determining whether there is a family history of diabetes. The second thing to determine, by measuring fasting triglyceride levels before and after starting an atypical antipsychotic, is whether atypical antipsychotics are causing dyslipidemia and increased

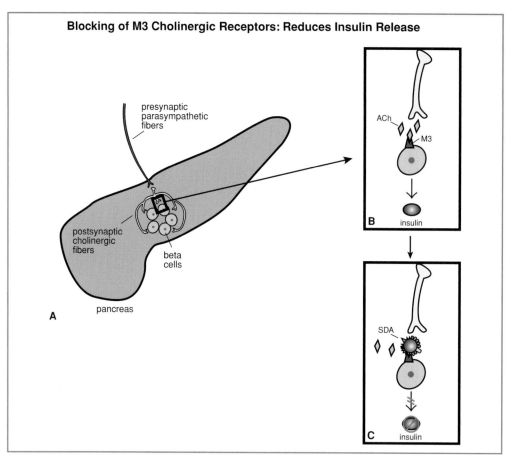

Blocking of M3 Cholinergic Receptors: Reduces Insulin Release

FIGURE 2-64A, B and C Blocking M3-cholinergic receptors reduces insulin release. (A) Insulin secretion is regulated in part by parasympathetic cholinergic neurons that synapse with pancreatic beta cells. (B) When acetylcholine (ACh) binds to muscarinic-3 (M3) receptors on pancreatic beta cells, this causes insulin secretion. (C) Thus, agents that block M3 receptors – such as certain atypical antipsychotics like olanzapine and clozapine – may reduce insulin release.

insulin resistance (Figure 2-66). If body mass index or fasting triglycerides increase significantly, a switch to a different antipsychotic that does not cause these problems should be considered (Figure 2-67). In patients who are obese, have dyslipidemia, and are in either a prediabetic or diabetic state, it is especially important to monitor blood pressure, fasting glucose, and waist circumference before and after initiating an atypical antipsychotic. Best practices are to monitor these parameters in anyone taking any atypical antipsychotic (Figure 2-67). In high-risk patients, it is especially important to be vigilant for DKA/HHS, and possibly to reduce that risk by maintaining such patients on an antipsychotic with lower cardiometabolic risk (Tables 2-3 and 2-4; Figure 2-67). In high-risk patients, especially those with pending or actual pancreatic beta cell failure as manifested by hyperinsulinemia, prediabetes, or diabetes, fasting glucose and other chemical and clinical parameters can be monitored to detect early signs of rare but potentially fatal DKA/HHS (Figure 2-66).

So, does a psychopharmacologist have to become an endocrinologist? The answer is no. The psychopharmacologist's metabolic tool kit is quite simple (Figure 2-68). It involves a flowchart that tracks perhaps as few as four parameters over time, with documentation

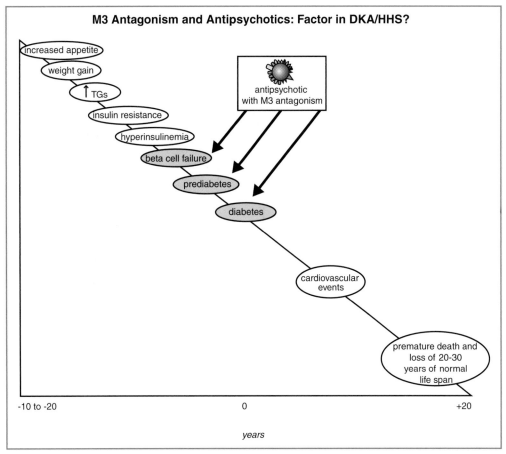

FIGURE 2-65 M3 antagonism and antipsychotics: factor in DKA/HHS? An atypical antipsychotic with muscarinic 3 (M3) antagonism could reduce insulin release by binding to M3 receptors on pancreatic beta cells. In patients with undiagnosed insulin resistance, prediabetes, or diabetes, this could potentially lead to diabetic ketoacidosis (DKA) or hyperglycemic hyperosmolar syndrome (HHS). However, not all patients have problems with insulin secretion when M3 receptors are blocked; additional mechanisms are likely to be important in the production of DKA/HHS by atypical antipsychotics.

being especially important before and after switches from one antipsychotic to another or as new risk factors evolve. These four parameters are weight (as body mass index), fasting triglycerides, fasting glucose, and blood pressure.

The management of patients at risk for cardiometabolic disease can be quite simple as well, although patients who have already developed dyslipidemia, hypertension, diabetes, and heart disease will likely require management of these problems by a medical specialist. However, the psychopharmacologist is left with a very simple set of options for managing patients with cardiometabolic risk who are taking an atypical antipsychotic (Figure 2-69). The major factors that determine whether such a patient progresses along the metabolic highway to premature death include those that are unmanageable (e.g., the patient's genetic makeup and age), those that are modestly manageable (e.g., change in lifestyle, such as diet, exercise, and stopping smoking), and those that are most manageable, namely the selection of antipsychotic and perhaps switching from one that is causing increased risk in a particular

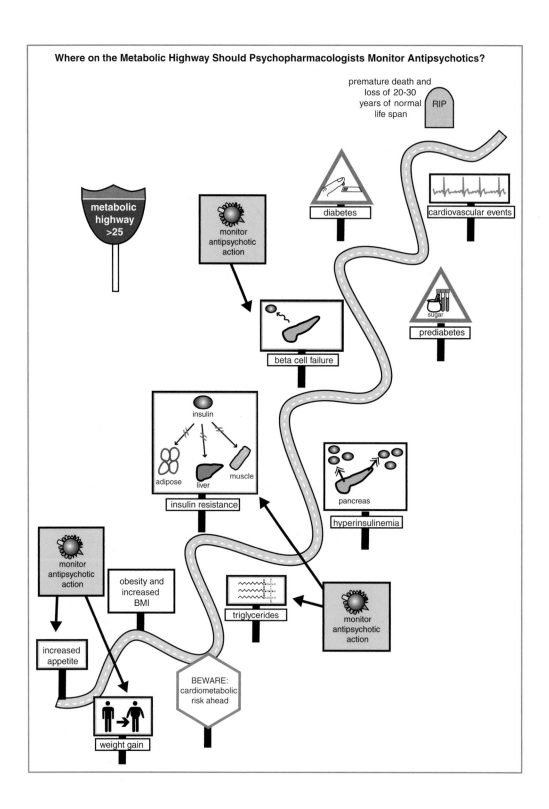

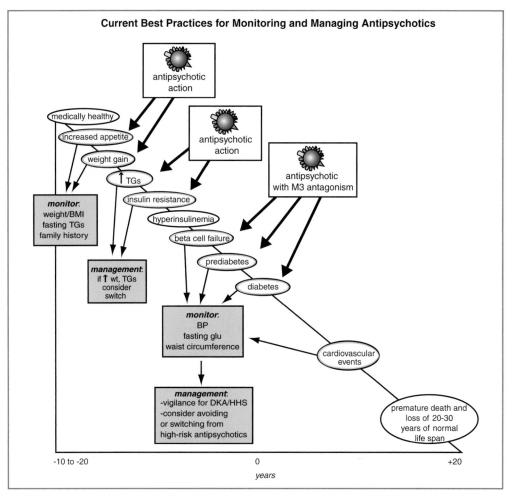

Current Best Practices for Monitoring and Managing Antipsychotics

antipsychotic action

medically healthy

increased appetite

weight gain

antipsychotic action

↑ TGs

insulin resistance

antipsychotic with M3 antagonism

monitor:
weight/BMI
fasting TGs
family history

hyperinsulinemia

beta cell failure

management:
if ↑ wt, TGs
consider
switch

prediabetes

diabetes

monitor:
BP
fasting glu
waist circumference

cardiovascular events

management:
-vigilance for DKA/HHS
-consider avoiding
or switching from
high-risk antipsychotics

premature death and
loss of 20-30
years of normal
life span

-10 to -20   0   +20

years

FIGURE 2-67 Current best practices for monitoring and managing antipsychotics. Monitoring should occur prior to the initiation of an antipsychotic, with baseline measurements including weight, body mass index (BMI), fasting triglyceride levels (TGs), and family history of diabetes. Weight, BMI, and fasting triglycerides should continue to be monitored throughout treatment. If patients do show an increase in weight or triglyceride levels, they may need to be switched to a different antipsychotic, adopt lifestyle changes, or both. For patients who are obese, have dyslipidemia, or are prediabetic or diabetic, it is important to monitor blood pressure, fasting glucose, and waist circumference both before and after starting an antipsychotic as well as to be vigilant for diabetic ketoacidosis (DKA) and hyperglycemic hyperosmolar syndrome (HHS). One may choose to avoid or switch from antipsychotics with higher risk of cardiometabolic effects.

FIGURE 2-66 Monitoring on the metabolic highway. Where on the metabolic highway should psychopharmacologists monitor antipsychotics? Key stages along the metabolic highway where antipsychotics can produce cardiometabolic risks are the places where the actions of these drugs should be monitored. Thus, there are at least three "on" ramps where the cardiometabolic risk of some atypical antipsychotics can enter the metabolic highway, and they are all shown here. First, increased appetite and weight gain can lead to elevated body mass index (BMI) and ultimately obesity. Thus, weight and BMI should be monitored here. Second, atypical antipsychotics can cause insulin resistance by an unknown mechanism; this can be detected by measuring fasting plasma triglyceride levels. Finally, atypical antipsychotics can cause sudden onset of diabetic ketoacidosis (DKA) or hyperglycemic hyperosmolar syndrome (HHS) by unknown mechanisms, possibly including blockade of M3-cholinergic receptors. This can be detected by informing patients of the symptoms of DKA/HHS and by measuring fasting glucose levels.

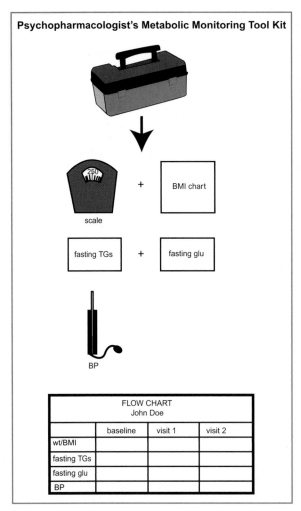

Psychopharmacologist's Metabolic Monitoring Tool Kit

scale + BMI chart

fasting TGs + fasting glu

BP

FLOW CHART John Doe			
	baseline	visit 1	visit 2
wt/BMI			
fasting TGs			
fasting glu			
BP			

FIGURE 2-68 Metabolic monitoring tool kit. The psychopharmacologist's metabolic monitoring tool kit includes items for tracking four major parameters: weight/body mass index, fasting triglycerides (TGs), fasting glucose, and blood pressure. These items are simply a flowchart that can appear at the beginning of a patient's chart with entries for each visit, a scale, a BMI chart to convert weight into BMI, a blood pressure cuff, and laboratory results for fasting triglycerides and fasting glucose.

patient to one that, on monitoring, demonstrates a reduced risk (Tables 2-2 through 2-4; Figure 2-69).

Sedation and antipsychotics

Antipsychotics are associated with sedation, and sedation has several potential mechanisms (Figures 2-70 and 2-71). Not only can blocking D2 receptors cause sedation, particularly at high doses that cause neurolepsis, but so can blocking M1-muscarinic cholinergic receptors, H1-histamine receptors, and alpha-1 adrenergic receptors (Figures 2-70 and 2-71). Dopamine, acetylcholine, histamine, and norepinephrine are all involved in arousal pathways (Figure 2-71), so it is not surprising that the blocking of one or more of these systems can lead to sedation. For our purposes, it is useful to point out that one can produce or avoid sedation by understanding the pharmacology of this clinical effect (Figures 2-70 and 2-71) and by knowing which drugs have such pharmacological properties and which do not (see later discussion of individual drugs and Figures 2-90 through 2-104).

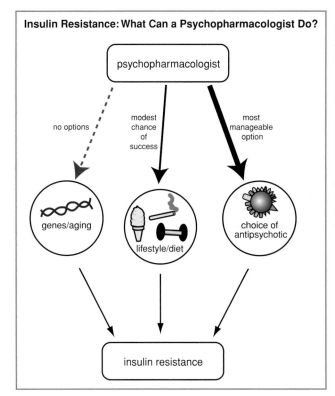

Insulin Resistance: What Can a Psychopharmacologist Do?

psychopharmacologist

no options

modest chance of success

most manageable option

genes/aging

lifestyle/diet

choice of antipsychotic

insulin resistance

FIGURE 2-69 Insulin resistance: what can a psychopharmacologist do? Several factors influence whether or not an individual develops insulin resistance, some of which are manageable by a psychopharmacologist and some of which are not. Unmanageable factors include genetic makeup and age, while items that are modestly manageable include lifestyle (e.g., diet, exercise, smoking). Psychopharmacologists exert their greatest influence on managing insulin resistance through selection of antipsychotics that either do or do not cause insulin resistance.

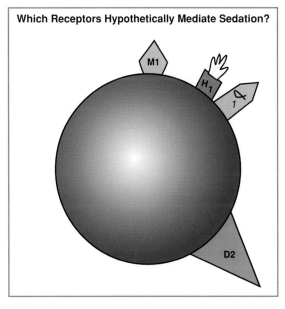

Which Receptors Hypothetically Mediate Sedation?

M1

H₁

1

D2

FIGURE 2-70 Which receptors hypothetically mediate sedation? Antagonism of D2 receptors, as well as of muscarinic-1, histamine-1, and alpha-1 adrenergic receptors, could hypothetically mediate sedation.

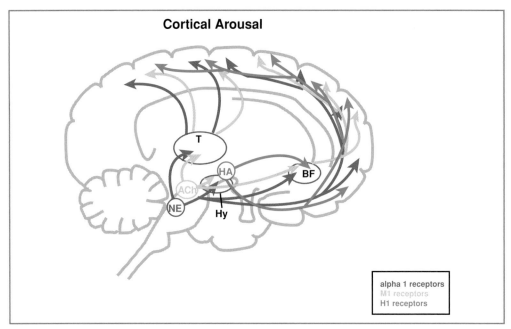

FIGURE 2-71 **Neurotransmitters of cortical arousal.** The neurotransmitters acetylcholine (ACh), histamine (HA), and norepinephrine (NE) are all involved in arousal pathways connecting neurotransmitter centers with the thalamus (T), hypothalamus (Hy), basal forebrain (BF), and cortex. Thus, pharmacological actions at their receptors could influence arousal. In particular, antagonism of muscarinic M1, histamine H1, and alpha-1 adrenergic receptors are all associated with sedating effects.

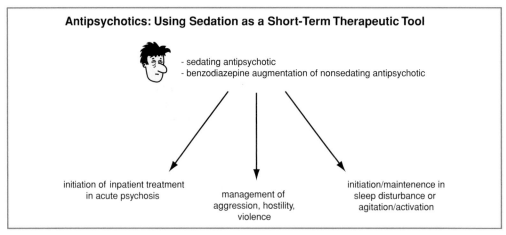

FIGURE 2-72 **Antipsychotics: Using sedation as a short term therapeutic tool.** Short-term, sedation can be beneficial for management of acute psychosis; aggression, hostility, or violence; sleep disturbances; or agitation/activation. This can be achieved with sedating antipsychotics or by augmentation with a benzodiazepine.

In some cases, sedation is a desired therapeutic effect, particularly early in treatment, during hospitalization, and when patients are aggressive, agitated, or needing sleep induction (Figure 2-72). This can be accomplished either with a sedating antipsychotic that has muscarinic, histaminic, and adrenergic blocking properties or by adding a sedating

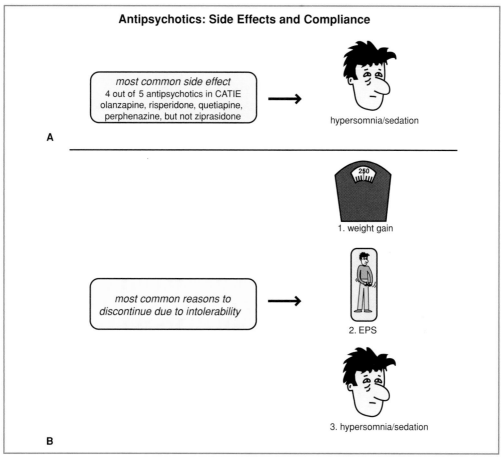

FIGURE 2-73A and B Antipsychotics, side effects and compliance. (**A**) Sedation is a common side effect of several antipsychotics, including many of the atypical antipsychotics, as shown in studies such as CATIE (Clinical Antipsychotic Trials of Intervention Effectiveness). (**B**) Long-term sedation may need to be avoided, as it is among the top three reasons for discontinuation due to intolerability, falling just behind weight gain and extrapyramidal symptoms (EPS).

benzodiazepine to any antipsychotic, especially those that are not sedating and lack these pharmacological properties (Figure 2-72).

In other cases, particularly for long-term treatment, sedation is generally a side effect to be avoided. Sedation is the most common side effect reported for many antipsychotics, especially those with a mixture of muscarinic, histaminic, and adrenergic blocking properties. Along with weight gain and EPS, sedation is one of the most common reasons for a patient to discontinue treatment with an antipsychotic drug (Figure 2-73). Furthermore, diminished arousal, sedation, and somnolence can lead to cognitive impairment, since cognitive functioning is mediated by these same pathways (Figure 2-71). When cognition is impaired, functional outcomes are compromised (Figures 2-74 through 2-77).

Pharmacological evidence suggests that the best long-term outcomes in schizophrenia result from adequate D2/5HT2A/5HT1A receptor occupancy, improving positive and especially negative and cognitive symptoms, rather than from nonspecific sedation resulting from muscarinic, histaminic, and adrenergic receptor blockade (Figures 2-74 through

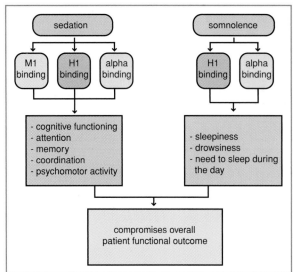

FIGURE 2-74 Sedation vs. somnolence. Sedation may be caused by antagonism of muscarinic M1, histamine H1, and/or alpha-1 adrenergic receptors. Sedation as a result of blocking these receptors may contribute to impaired cognitive functioning, attention, memory, and coordination, which in turn could affect overall patient functioning. Somnolence may be distinct from sedation and become manifest more as sleepiness, drowsiness, and the need to sleep during the day. These symptoms may be regulated by H1 and alpha 1 adrenergic receptors and can also affect overall patient functioning.

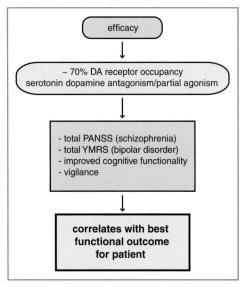

FIGURE 2-75 Efficacy profile. The best long-term outcomes in schizophrenia occur when patients experience relief not only from positive symptoms but also from affective, cognitive, and negative symptoms. From a pharmacological perspective, this can be achieved through blocking approximately 70 percent of D2 receptors in the nucleus accumbens plus antagonism/partial agonism of D2, serotonin-2A, and serotonin-1A receptors in other key brain regions and not from interaction with histamine H1, muscarinic M1, or alpha-1 adrenergic receptors. PANSS, Positive and Negative Symptom Scale; YMRS, Young Mania Rating Scale.

2-76). Thus, if sedation and somnolence cause cognitive impairment and cognitive impairment is linked to poor patient outcomes, sedation and somnolence may also be linked to poor patient outcomes (Figure 2-76). On the other hand, if optimum D2/5HT2A/5HT1A receptor actions are combined with levels of muscarinic, histaminic, and adrenergic receptor blockade that do not cause sedation, perhaps the best patient outcomes will be achieved (Figure 2-75 through 2-77). Sometimes this is easier said than done, but drug selection based on desired pharmacological profile can result in managing sedation in a clinically useful manner while obtaining the best patient outcomes (Figure 2-77).

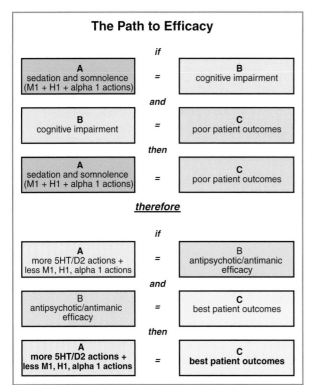

The Path to Efficacy

if

| A
sedation and somnolence
(M1 + H1 + alpha 1 actions) | = | B
cognitive impairment |

and

| B
cognitive impairment | = | C
poor patient outcomes |

then

| A
sedation and somnolence
(M1 + H1 + alpha 1 actions) | = | C
poor patient outcomes |

therefore

if

| A
more 5HT/D2 actions +
less M1, H1, alpha 1 actions | = | B
antipsychotic/antimanic
efficacy |

and

| B
antipsychotic/antimanic
efficacy | = | C
best patient outcomes |

then

| A
more 5HT/D2 actions +
less M1, H1, alpha 1 actions | = | C
best patient outcomes |

FIGURE 2-76 The path to efficacy. If sedation and somnolence (mediated by M1, H1, and alpha-1 actions) lead to cognitive impairment and cognitive impairment is associated with poor patient outcomes, sedation and somnolence (mediated by M1, H1, and alpha-1) would therefore be related to poor patient outcomes. On the other hand, if serotonergic and dopaminergic actions with minimal effects on M1, H1, and alpha-1 receptors are related to antipsychotic and antimanic efficacy and if antipsychotic/ antimanic efficacy is associated with good patient outcomes, an antipsychotic with a serotonergic and dopaminergic profile but without actions at M1, H1, or alpha-1 receptors should lead to good patient outcomes.

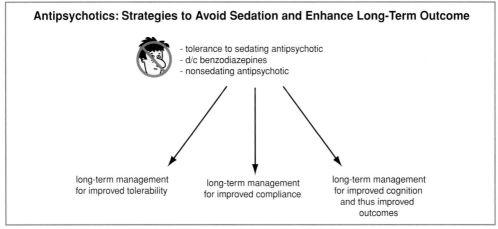

Antipsychotics: Strategies to Avoid Sedation and Enhance Long-Term Outcome

- tolerance to sedating antipsychotic
- d/c benzodiazepines
- nonsedating antipsychotic

long-term management for improved tolerability

long-term management for improved compliance

long-term management for improved cognition and thus improved outcomes

FIGURE 2-77 Antipsychotics: Strategies to avoid sedation and enhance long-term outcome. Achieving the best long-term outcomes in schizophrenia may require avoiding long-term sedation. For patients whose treatment was initiated with a nonsedating antipsychotic but who received an adjunct benzodiazepine, this may mean discontinuing the benzodiazepine. Some patients initiated on a sedating antipsychotic may develop tolerance to the sedating side effects and not require treatment adjustment; however, others may need to be switched to a nonsedating agent.

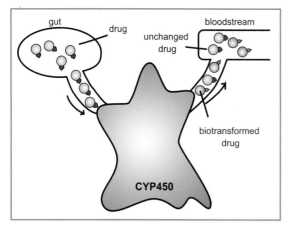

FIGURE 2-78 CYP450. The cytochrome P450 (CYP450) enzyme system mediates how the body metabolizes many drugs, including antipsychotics. The CYP450 enzyme in the gut wall or liver converts the drug into a biotransformed product in the bloodstream. After passing through the gut wall and liver (left), the drug will exist partly as unchanged drug and partly as biotransformed drug (right).

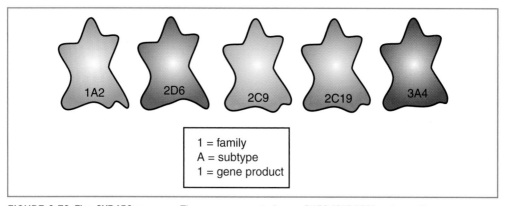

1 = family
A = subtype
1 = gene product

FIGURE 2-79 Five CYP450 enzymes. There are many cytochrome P450 (CYP450) systems; these are classified according to family, subtype, and gene product. Five of the most important are shown here, and include CYP450 1A2, 2D6, 2C9, 2C19, and 3A4.

Antipsychotic pharmacokinetics

Pharmacokinetics is the study of how the body acts on drugs, especially to absorb, distribute, metabolize, and excrete them. These pharmacokinetic actions are mediated through the hepatic and gut drug metabolizing system known as the cytochrome P450 (CYP450) enzyme system. The CYP450 enzymes and the **pharmacokinetic** actions they represent must be contrasted with the **pharmacodynamic** actions of the antipsychotics discussed extensively so far in this chapter. Although most of this book deals with the **pharmacodynamics** of psychopharmacological agents, especially how drugs act on the brain, the following section will discuss the **pharmacokinetics** of antipsychotics, or how the body acts on these drugs.

Figure 2-78 shows how an antipsychotic is absorbed and delivered through the gut wall to the liver to be biotransformed so that it can be excreted from the body. Specifically, CYP450 enzymes in the gut wall or liver convert the drug substrate into a biotransformed product in the bloodstream. After passing through the gut wall and liver, the drug exists partially as unchanged drug and partially as biotransformed product (Figure 2-78).

There are several known CYP450 systems. Five of the most important enzymes for antidepressant drug metabolism are shown in Figure 2-79. There are over thirty known

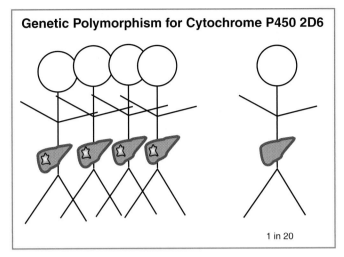

Genetic Polymorphism for Cytochrome P450 2D6

1 in 20

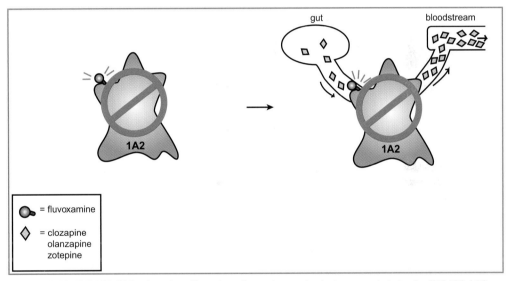

gut

bloodstream

1A2

1A2

= fluvoxamine

= clozapine
olanzapine
zotepine

FIGURE 2-81 CYP450 1A2 substrates. Clozapine, olanzapine, and zotepine are substrates for CYP450 1A2. When these antipsychotics are given with an inhibitor of this enzyme, such as the antidepressant fluvoxamine, their plasma levels can rise.

CYP450 enzymes and probably many more awaiting discovery and classification. Not all individuals have all the same CYP450 enzymes. In such cases, the enzyme is said to be polymorphic. For example, about 5 to 10 percent of Caucasians are poor metabolizers via the enzyme CYP450 2D6 (Figure 2-80). They must metabolize drugs by alternative routes, which may not be as efficient as the CYP450 2D6 route. Another CYP450 enzyme, 2C19, has reduced activity in approximately 20 percent of Japanese and Chinese individuals and in 3 to 5 percent of Caucasians.

CYP450 1A2. One CYP450 enzyme of relevance to antipsychotics is 1A2 (Figures 2-81 and 2-82). Three atypical antipsychotics are substrates for 1A2, namely olanzapine, clozapine, and zotepine. This means that when they are given concomitantly with

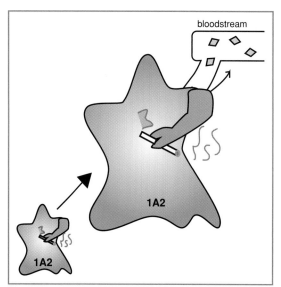

FIGURE 2-82 CYP450 1A2 and smoking.
Cigarette smoking, quite common among schizophrenic patients, can induce the enzyme CYP450 1A2 and lower the concentration of drugs metabolized by this enzyme, such as olanzapine, clozapine, and zotepine. Smokers may also require higher doses of these drugs than nonsmokers.

bloodstream

1A2

1A2

an inhibitor of this enzyme, such as the antidepressant fluvoxamine, their levels may rise (Figure 2-81). Although this may not be particularly important clinically for olanzapine (possibly causing slightly increased sedation), it could potentially raise plasma levels sufficiently in the case of clozapine or zotepine to increase the risk of seizures. Thus, the dose of clozapine or zotepine may need to be lowered when it is administered with fluvoxamine, or another antidepressant may need to be chosen.

On the other hand, when an inducer of 1A2 is given concomitantly with any of the three antipsychotic substrates for 1A2, their levels may fall. This happens when a patient begins to smoke, because smoking induces 1A2, and this would cause levels of olanzapine and clozapine to fall (Figure 2-82). Theoretically this might cause patients stabilized on an antipsychotic dose to relapse if the drug levels fell too low. Also, cigarette smokers may require higher doses of these atypical antipsychotics than nonsmokers.

CYP 2C9. The new DPA (dopamine partial agonist) bifeprunox is a substrate of 2C9, and its levels are increased by coadministration of a 2C9 inhibitor such as fluconazole.

CYP 2D6. Another CYP450 enzyme of importance to atypical antipsychotic drugs is the enzyme 2D6. Risperidone, clozapine, olanzapine, and aripiprazole are all substrates for this enzyme (Figure 2-83). Risperidone's metabolite is paliperidone, itself recently approved as a new atypical antipsychotic (Figure 2-84). Paliperidone itself thus bypasses the 2D6 enzyme, is not a substrate for 2D6, and is therefore not affected by alterations in the activity of the 2D6 enzyme, unlike its precursor risperidone (Figures 2-83 and 2-84).

Several antidepressants are inhibitors of 2D6 and thus can raise the levels of the atypical antipsychotics that are substrates of 2D6 (Figure 2-85). For risperidone, this shifts the balance away from formation of the active metabolite paliperidone, which could potentially increase EPS. Theoretically, the dose of olanzapine, clozapine, or aripiprazole may have to be lowered when given with an antidepressant that blocks 2D6, although this is not often necessary in practice.

CYP 3A4. This enzyme metabolizes several atypical antipsychotics including clozapine, quetiapine, ziprasidone, sertindole, aripiprazole, zotepine, and bifeprunox (Figure 2-86). Several psychotropic drugs are weak inhibitors of this enzyme, including the

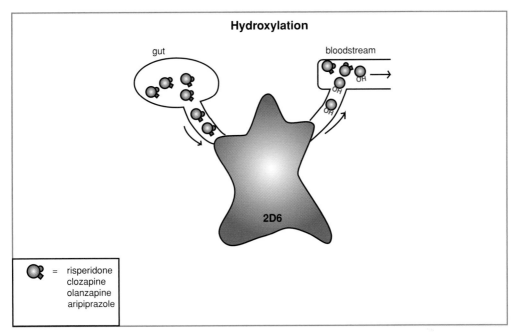

Hydroxylation

gut

bloodstream

2D6

= risperidone
clozapine
olanzapine
aripiprazole

FIGURE 2-83 CYP450 2D6 substrates. Several atypical antipsychotics are substrates for CYP450 2D6, including risperidone, clozapine, olanzapine, and aripiprazole. 2D6 often hydroxylates drug substrates.

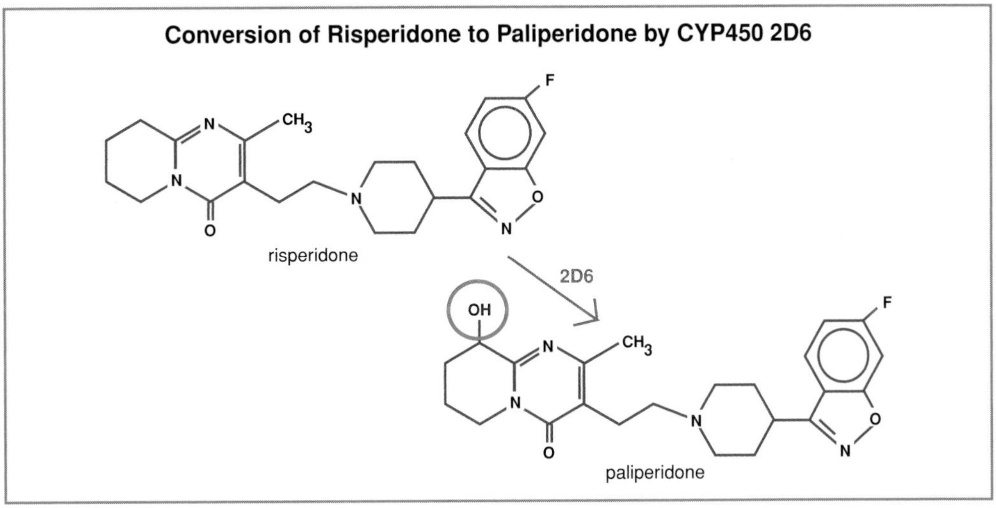

Conversion of Risperidone to Paliperidone by CYP450 2D6

risperidone

2D6

paliperidone

FIGURE 2-84 Paliperidone. Conversion of risperidone to paliperidone by CYP450 2D6. Risperidone is converted to the active metabolite paliperidone by the enzyme CYP450 2D6. Paliperidone is now available as an antipsychotic.

antidepressants fluvoxamine, nefazodone, and the active metabolite of fluoxetine, norfluoxetine. Several nonpsychotropic drugs are powerful inhibitors of 3A4, including ketoconazole (antifungal), protease inhibitors (for AIDS/HIV) and erythromycin (antibiotic). For atypical antipsychotics that are substrates of 3A4, the clinical implication is that concomitant administration with a 3A4 inhibitor may require dosage reduction of the atypical antipsychotic (Figure 2-87).

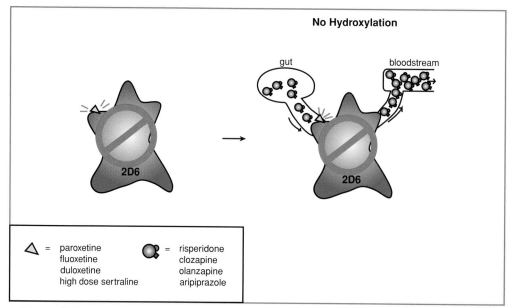

FIGURE 2-85 CYP450 2D6 inhibitors. Several antidepressants are inhibitors of CYP450 2D6 and could theoretically raise the levels of 2D6 substrates such as risperidone, clozapine, olanzapine, and aripiprazole. However, this is not usually clinically significant.

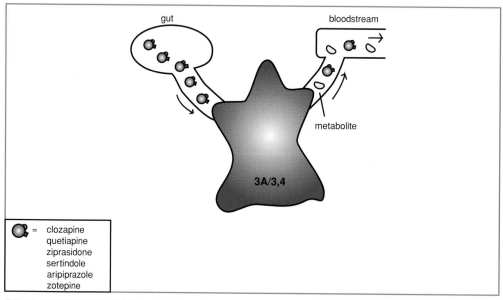

FIGURE 2-86 CYP450 3 A/3,4 substrates. Several atypical antipsychotics are substrates for CYP450 3A4, including clozapine, quetiapine, ziprasidone, sertindole, aripiprazole, and zotepine.

Drugs can not only be substrates for a CYP450 enzyme or inhibitors of a P450 enzyme but also inducers of a CYP450 enzyme, thereby increasing the activity of that enzyme. An example of this is the anticonvulsant and mood stabilizer carbamazepine, which induces the activity of 3A4 (Figure 2-88). Since mood stabilizers may frequently be mixed with atypical antipsychotics, it is possible that carbamazepine may be added to the regimen of a

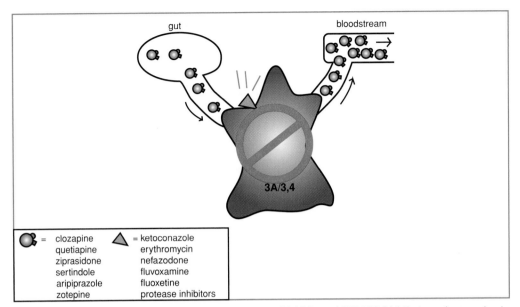

FIGURE 2-87 CYP450 3 A/3,4 inhibitors. There are several inhibitors of CYP450 3A4 that may increase levels of those atypical antipsychotics that are substrates for 3A4. The inhibitors for 3A4 are shown here, as are the atypical antipsychotics that are substrates for 3A4.

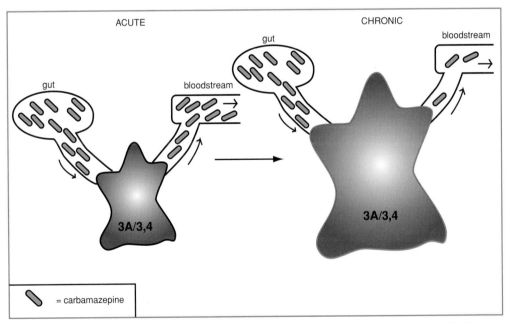

FIGURE 2-88 CYP450 3A4 induced by carbamazepine. The enzyme CYP450 3A4 can be induced by the anticonvulsant and mood stabilizer carbamazepine. This would lead to increased metabolism of substrates for 3A4 (e.g., clozapine, quetiapine, ziprasidone, sertindole, aripiprazole, and zotepine) and may therefore require higher doses of these agents when given concomitantly with carbamazepine.

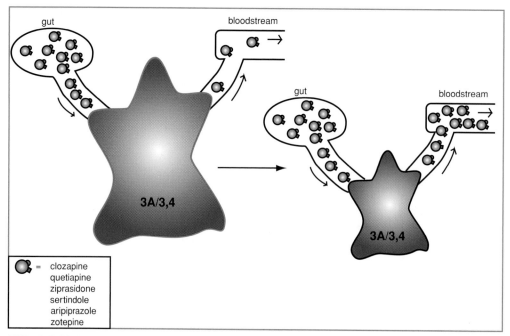

FIGURE 2-89 CYP450 3A4 and carbamazepine discontinuation. If carbamazepine, which induces CYP450 3A4, is discontinued in a patient who is receiving an atypical antipsychotic that is a substrate for this same enzyme (e.g., clozapine, quetiapine, ziprasidone, sertindole, aripiprazole, and zotepine), the doses of these antipsychotics may need to be reduced, because the autoinduction of 3A4 by carbamazepine will reverse over time once it is discontinued.

patient previously stabilized on clozapine, quetiapine, ziprasidone, sertindole, aripiprazole, or zotepine. If so, the doses of these atypical antipsychotics may need to be increased over time to compensate for the induction of 3A4 caused by carbamazepine. On the other hand, if carbamazepine is stopped in a patient receiving one of these atypical antipsychotics, their doses may need to be reduced, because the autoinduction of 3A4 by carbamazepine will reverse over time (Figure 2-89).

This discussion of antipsychotic pharmacokinetics is not comprehensive but merely conceptual, leaving out many important details the prescriber will need to know. In this rapidly evolving area of therapeutics, the only way to keep up is to continually consult updated standard reference materials on drug interactions and the specific dosing implications that such interactions cause (such as S.M. Stahl, *Essential Psychopharmacology: The Prescriber's Guide*, a companion to this book). In summary, drug interactions may potentially require dosage adjustment of one of the drugs. A few combinations must be strictly avoided. Many drug interactions are statistically but not clinically significant. By following the principles outlined here, the skilled practitioner and prescriber of antipsychotic agents must learn whether any given drug interaction is clinically relevant.

Pharmacological properties of individual antipsychotics

The pharmacological properties hypothetically linked to what makes an antipsychotic atypical have been extensively discussed earlier in this chapter. These concepts are necessary for explaining some of the atypical clinical actions of several atypical antipsychotics, but they are not sufficient for explaining all of the clinical properties of these unique therapeutic agents. Thus, even though atypical antipsychotics do share some key pharmacological properties

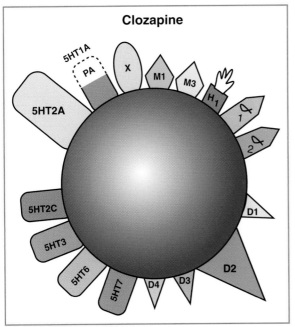

Clozapine

FIGURE 2-90 Clozapine's pharmacological icon. The most prominent binding properties of clozapine are represented here; this is perhaps one of the most complex binding portfolios in all of psychopharmacology. Clozapine's binding properties vary greatly with technique and species and from one laboratory to another. This icon portrays a qualitative consensus of current thinking about the binding properties of clozapine, which are constantly being revised and updated. In addition to serotonin 2A/D2 antagonism (SDA properties), at least thirteen other pharmacological actions have been identified for clozapine. It is unknown which of these contribute to clozapine's special efficacy or to its unique side effects.

with each other, in many other ways they also have distinctive pharmacological properties that differentiate one atypical antipsychotic from another. Such pharmacological distinctions are candidates for explaining the widely observed differences in tolerability or efficacy of these agents for individual patients. That is, many patients will tolerate one atypical antipsychotic better than another or will respond to one better than to another. The reasons for these observations remain mysteries and are difficult to prove in large randomized multicenter trials, yet differences are commonly observed in clinical practice.

What follows are some ideas and some conjectures about what makes one atypical antipsychotic different from another on the basis of known pharmacological distinctions of one drug versus another. Here we will review some of the differences among fifteen selected antipsychotic agents based both on the art and the science of psychopharmacology. Further details of the individual drugs are available in the companion *Prescriber's Guide* (S. M. Stahl, *Essential Psychopharmacology: The Prescriber's Guide*) and other standard references. The pharmacological properties represented in the icons shown in the next section are conceptual and not quantitative, can differ from one laboratory to another, and evolve over time. The point is really that no two atypical antipsychotics have exactly the same pharmacological binding profiles even though some of their properties at dopamine and serotonin receptors overlap. These distinctive properties may be worth noting in order to match the best antipsychotic agent to the individual patient.

Clozapine. Clozapine, a serotonin 2A/dopamine D2 antagonist, or SDA (Figure 2-90), is considered to be the "prototypical" atypical antipsychotic and has one of the most complex pharmacological profiles of any of the atypical antipsychotics. Clozapine was the first antipsychotic to be recognized as atypical and thus to cause few if any extrapyramidal side effects, not to cause tardive dyskinesia, and not to elevate prolactin. Despite its complex pharmacology, these atypical properties were linked to the presence of serotonin-2A antagonism added to the dopamine-D2 antagonism of conventional antipsychotics.

Clozapine is the one atypical antipsychotic that is recognized as being particularly effective when conventional antipsychotic agents have failed and is thus the "gold standard" for efficacy in schizophrenia. It is unknown what pharmacological property accounts for this level of efficacy but it is unlikely to be simply serotonin 2A antagonism, since clozapine can show greater efficacy than other atypical antipsychotics that share this pharmacological property. Although patients treated with clozapine may occasionally experience an "awakening" (in the Oliver Sachs sense), characterized by return to a near normal level of cognitive, interpersonal, and vocational functioning and not just significant improvement in positive symptoms of psychosis, this is unfortunately rare. The fact that it can be observed at all, however, gives hope to the possibility that a state of wellness might some day be achieved in schizophrenia by the right mix of pharmacological mechanisms. Awakenings have been observed on rare occasions in association with treatment with other atypical antipsychotics but almost never in association with conventional antipsychotic treatment.

Clozapine is also the only antipsychotic that has been documented to reduce the risk of suicide in schizophrenia. It can be especially useful in quelling violence and aggression in difficult cases and may actually reduce the severity of tardive dyskinesia, especially over long treatment intervals. Although clozapine is certainly an SDA, the mechanism of its apparently enhanced efficacy profile compared to other antipsychotics remains the topic of vigorous debate.

Clozapine is also the only antipsychotic associated with the risk, in 0.5 to 2 percent of patients, of developing a life-threatening and occasionally fatal complication called agranulocytosis. Because of this, patients must have their blood counts monitored for as long as they are treated. Clozapine also poses an increased risk of seizures, especially at high doses. It can be very sedating, can cause excessive salivation, and is associated with an increased risk of myocarditis as well as the greatest degree of weight gain and possibly the greatest cardiometabolic risk among the antipsychotics. Thus, clozapine may have the greatest efficacy but also the most side effects among the atypical antipsychotics.

Because of these side-effect risks, clozapine is not generally considered to be a first-line treatment but is used when other antipsychotics fail. The mechanism of clozapine's ability to cause agranulocytosis, myocarditis, and seizures is entirely unknown, although the weight gain may be associated with its blockade of both H1-histamine and 5HT2C receptors (see Table 2-2 and Figures 2-58, 2-59, 2-61, 2-66, 2-67, and 2-90). Sedation is probably linked to clozapine's potent antagonism of M1-muscarinic, H1-histaminic, and alpha-1 adrenergic receptors (Figures 2-70, 2-71, and 2-90). Clozapine is among the antipsychotics most notable for increasing cardiometabolic risks (Table 2-3), including increases in fasting plasma triglyceride levels and increases in insulin resistance by an unknown but postulated pharmacological mechanism (receptor X in Figures 2-58, 2-62, 2-63, 2-66, 2-67, and 2-90). Finally, clozapine may rarely cause a sudden and life-threatening hyperglycemic hyperosmolar syndrome/diabetic ketoacidosis, possibly with M3 cholinergic antagonism being a factor, although the importance of this mechanism is still unproven (Figures 2-58, 2-64, 2-65, 2-66, 2-67, and 2-90).

Olanzapine. Although this agent has a chemical structure related to that of clozapine and is also an SDA, olanzapine is more potent than clozapine and has several differentiating pharmacological (Figure 2-91) and clinical features. Olanzapine is atypical in that it generally does not cause EPS, not only at moderate antipsychotic doses but usually even at higher ones. Olanzapine lacks the extreme sedating properties of clozapine but can be somewhat sedating in some patients, as it does have antagonist properties at M1-muscarinic, H1-histaminic, and alpha-1 adrenergic receptors (Figure 2-91). Olanzapine does not often raise

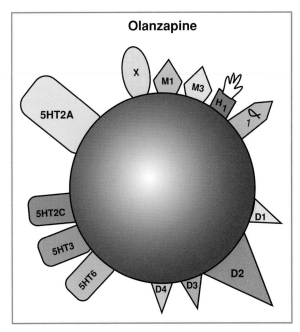

FIGURE 2-91 Olanzapine. Olanzapine's pharmacological icon, portraying a qualitative consensus of current thinking about the binding properties of this drug. It has a complex pharmacology overlapping yet different from that of clozapine. As with all atypical antipsychotics discussed in this chapter, binding properties vary greatly with technique and from one laboratory to another; they are constantly being revised and updated. In addition to SDA properties, 5HT2C antagonist properties may contribute to olanzapine's efficacy for mood and cognitive symptoms, although together with its H1-antihistamine properties could also contribute to olanzapine's propensity to cause weight gain.

prolactin levels. It is consistently associated with weight gain (Table 2-2), perhaps because of its antihistamine and 5HT2C antagonist properties (Figures 2-59 and 2-91). It ranks among the antipsychotics with the greatest known cardiometabolic risks (Table 2-3), as it robustly increases fasting triglyceride levels and increases insulin resistance by an unknown pharmacological mechanism postulated to be active for some atypical antipsychotics at least in some patients (receptor X in Figures 2-58, 2-62, 2-63, 2-66, 2-67, and 2-91). Olanzapine is also associated rarely with a sudden and life-threatening hyperglycemic hyperosmolar syndrome/diabetic ketoacidosis, possibly with M3 cholinergic antagonism being a factor, although, as for clozapine, the importance of this mechanism is still unproven (Figures 2-58, 2-64, 2-65, 2-66, 2-67, and 2-90).

Olanzapine tends to be used in higher doses in clinical practice than originally studied and approved for marketing, since there is the sense that higher doses might be associated not only with greater efficacy (i.e., improvement of clinical symptoms) but also with greater effectiveness (i.e., clinical outcome based on the balance of safety and efficacy) than moderate or low doses. Ongoing studies also show that olanzapine improves mood not only in schizophrenia but also in bipolar disorder and in treatment-resistant depression, particularly when combined with antidepressants such as fluoxetine. Perhaps the 5HT2C antagonist properties of olanzapine (Figure 2-91), especially when combined with the 5HT2C antagonist properties of the antidepressant fluoxetine, may explain some aspects of olanzapine's apparent efficacy for affective and cognitive symptoms.

For patients with significant weight gain or those who develop significant cardiometabolic risks, such as dyslipidemia (elevated fasting triglycerides) or diabetes, olanzapine may be considered a second-line agent. Olanzapine can, however, be considered an appropriate choice for patients when agents with a lower propensity for weight gain or cardiometabolic disturbances (Tables 2-2, 2-3, and 2-4) fail to achieve sufficient efficacy.

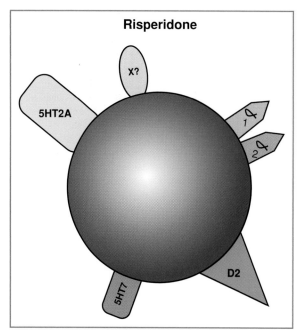

FIGURE 2-92 Risperidone. Risperidone's pharmacological icon, portraying a qualitative consensus of current thinking about the binding properties of this drug. Among the atypical antipsychotics, it has one of the simplest pharmacological profiles and comes closest to a serotonin-dopamine antagonist (SDA). As with all atypical antipsychotics discussed in this chapter, binding properties vary greatly with technique and from one laboratory to another; they are constantly being revised and updated. Alpha-2 antagonist properties may contribute to efficacy for depression, but this can be diminished by simultaneous alpha-1 antagonist properties, which can also contribute to orthostatic hypotension and sedation.

The decision to use any atypical antipsychotic requires the monitoring not only of efficacy but also risks, including cardiometabolic risks. The decision to use any particular agent is a trade-off between risks and benefits and must be determined for each individual patient and each individual drug.

Olanzapine is one of three atypical antipsychotics with an intramuscular dosage formulation for parenteral and emergent use and is also available as an oral disintegrating tablet.

Risperidone. This agent has a different chemical structure and a considerably simpler pharmacological profile than clozapine (i.e., risperidone is mostly an SDA) (Figure 2-92). Risperidone has atypical properties especially at lower doses but can become more "conventional" at high doses in that EPS can occur if the dose is too high. Risperidone thus has favored uses not only in schizophrenia and bipolar mania at moderate doses but also for "off-label" use in conditions where low doses of conventional antipsychotics have been used in the past, as for children and adolescents with psychotic disorders and for elderly patients with psychosis, agitation, and behavioral disturbances associated with dementia. Risperidone is the only agent with a pediatric approved use, and that is for treatment of irritability associated with autistic disorder in children and adolescents (ages 5 to 16), bipolar disorder (ages 10 to 17), and schizophrenia (ages 13 to 17). On the other hand, no antipsychotic is approved for psychosis associated with dementia, even though there is significant "off label" use of antipsychotics in general and risperidone in particular for psychosis and agitation associated with dementia. This occurs despite the fact that elderly patients with dementia-related psychosis treated with any atypical antipsychotic as compared with placebo are at increased risk of death, even though that overall risk is low. Obviously the risks versus benefits must be carefully weighed for each patient prior to prescribing an atypical antipsychotic for any use.

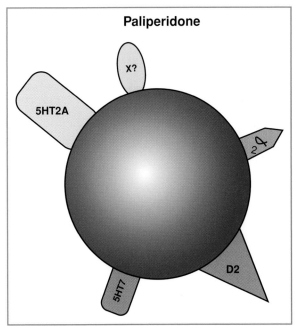

Paliperidone

FIGURE 2-93 Paliperidone. The pharmacological icon for paliperidone, the active metabolite of risperidone, is shown here. Paliperidone shares many pharmacological properties with risperidone but has less potent alpha-1 antagonist potency. This icon represents a qualitative consensus of current thinking about the binding properties of this drug; however, binding properties vary greatly with technique and from one laboratory to another. The greater prominence of alpha-2 antagonist actions suggests possible advantages for mood symptoms.

Risperidone is the only atypical antipsychotic available in a long-term depot injectable formulation lasting for 2 weeks. Such dosage formulations may improve compliance, and if compliance is enhanced, may lead to better long-term outcomes. There is also an orally disintegrating tablet of risperidone.

Many studies show that risperidone is a highly effective agent for positive symptoms of schizophrenia as well as for symptoms of mania in bipolar disorder, and it also improves negative symptoms of schizophrenia better than conventional antipsychotics. Although atypical in terms of reduced EPS, risperidone does raise prolactin levels. There is less weight gain with risperidone than with some other atypical antipsychotic agents (Table 2-2), perhaps because it does not potently block histamine-1 receptors (Figures 2-59 and 2-92), but weight gain is still a problem for some patients who take risperidone, especially children. There may also be less cardiometabolic risk with risperidone than with some other atypical antipsychotic agents (Table 2-3), but since it may increase insulin resistance and fasting triglycerides in some patients (Table 2-3), it may act by the postulated pharmacological mechanism discussed for clozapine and olanzapine (receptor X and Figures 2-58, 2-62, 2-63, 2-66, 2-67, and 2-92), at least in some patients. Although risperidone may also be associated rarely with sudden and life-threatening hyperglycemic hyperosmolar syndrome/diabetic ketoacidosis, it does not bind to M3 cholinergic receptors (Figures 2-58, 2-64, 2-65, 2-66, 2-67, and 2-92).

Paliperidone. Paliperidone, the active metabolite of risperidone, is also known as 9-hydroxy-risperidone and is an SDA (Figure 2-84 and 2-93). Unlike risperidone, the orally administered form of paliperidone is a sustained-release formulation, which means that it has to be taken only once daily (risperidone must sometimes be taken twice daily due to its shorter half-life), may require less dosage titration, and may have lower peak-dose plasma levels and thus lower EPS and sedation compared to risperidone. A depot palmitate formulation for long-term use of 4 weeks or more is in development as well.

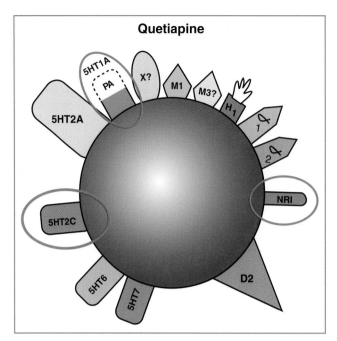

FIGURE 2-94 Quetiapine. Quetiapine's pharmacological icon, portraying a qualitative consensus of current thinking about the binding properties of this drug. It has a unique pharmacological profile, different from those of all other atypical antipsychotics. As with all atypical antipsychotics discussed in this chapter, binding properties vary greatly with technique and from one laboratory to another; they are constantly being revised and updated. Quetiapine's prominent H1-antagonist properties probably contribute to its ability to enhance sleep, and this may contribute as well to its ability to improve sleep disturbances in bipolar and unipolar depression as well as in anxiety disorders. However, this property can also contribute to daytime sedation, especially combined with M1-antimuscarinic and alpha-1 adrenergic antagonist properties. Recently, a potentially important active metabolite of quetiapine, norquetiapine, has been identified; in addition to some of the pharmacological properties noted here for the parent compound, norquetiapine may contribute additional actions at 5HT1A receptors and unique actions as a norepinephrine (NE) reuptake inhibitor (NRI) or NE transport inhibitor (NET) as well as antagonist actions at 5HT2C receptors (see red circles for unique actions contributed by the active metabolite norquetiapine). 5HT1A partial agonist actions, NET inhibition, and 5HT2C antagonist actions may all contribute to mood-improving properties as well as to cognitive enhancement by quetiapine. However, 5HT2C antagonist actions combined with H1 antagonist actions may contribute to weight gain.

Paliperidone's efficacy may be linked in part to alpha-2 antagonist properties, specifically for improving depression (Figure 2-93), especially since it may have less potent alpha-1 than alpha-2 antagonist potency. Risperidone also has alpha-2 antagonist properties, but its somewhat more potent alpha-1 antagonist properties can not only potentially mitigate antidepressant actions but also cause more orthostatic hypotension, particularly on dose initiation, compared to paliperidone.

Weight gain, insulin resistance, and diabetes may be associated with the use of paliperidone, as may elevations of plasma prolactin, with much the same risk as that of risperidone. Paliperidone has not been shown to bind to M3 cholinergic receptors.

Quetiapine. Quetiapine also has a chemical structure related to clozapine and is an SDA, but it has several differentiating pharmacological properties (Figure 2-94). In addition, norquetiapine – an active metabolite that has unique pharmacological properties which may contribute to quetiapine's overall pharmacological profile – has recently been characterized (Figure 2-94).

Quetiapine is "very atypical" in that it causes virtually no EPS at any dose; neither does it cause elevations in prolactin, perhaps related to its particularly rapid dissociation from D2 receptors (discussed above and illustrated in Figures 2-39 through 2-44). Thus, quetiapine tends to be the preferred atypical antipsychotic for patients with Parkinson's disease and psychosis. When dosed adequately, quetiapine is also highly effective in the treatment of schizophrenia and bipolar mania, and is the first atypical antipsychotic proven effective as a monotherapy for the treatment of the depressed phase of bipolar disorder. Quetiapine's 5HT1A partial agonist properties and those of its active metabolite norquetiapine may contribute to the overall efficacy of this agent for treating disorders of mood and cognition (Figure 2-94). In addition, norquetiapine can block the norepinephrine transporter (NET) (Figure 2-94), which would theoretically enhance norepinephrine (and dopamine) levels as do other known antidepressants and cognitive enhancers with this mechanism. Furthermore, norquetiapine can block 5HT2C receptors (Figure 2-94), which should enhance the release of both norepinephrine and dopamine and contribute to antidepressant action and cognitive improvement. An oral controlled-release formulation is now available that may not only enhance the duration of action of quetiapine and reduce its peak-dose actions, such as sedation, but also enhance the formation of the active metabolite norquetiapine and its contributions to the overall actions of this agent.

Although an agent with a short half-life that was originally studied with thrice-daily administration, quetiapine is clearly effective with once-daily administration for many patients, particularly at night, so that the sedating H1-antihistamine actions treat insomnia and wear off by morning, thus preventing daytime sedation. Quetiapine proves the point discussed earlier in this chapter that antipsychotics may not need to be administered often enough to keep D2 receptors occupied by drug for 24 hours a day. As mentioned earlier, this may be due to the possibility that continuous receptor occupancy may not be required for therapeutic actions but may in fact contribute to the undesired side effects. Indeed, what may be required for therapeutic efficacy may be akin to "ringing a bell" by clanging the receptor just once a day. The receptor continues to resonate long after the atypical antipsychotic hits it. That clearly is the case for the use of quetiapine in general and for its particular use as an agent to treat the depressed phase of bipolar disorder.

Quetiapine can cause weight gain (Table 2-2), particularly when given in moderate to high doses, as it blocks histamine-1 receptors (Figures 2-59 and 2-94). The 5HT2C actions of its active metabolite norquetiapine may contribute to weight gain at moderate to high doses of quetiapine (Figure 2-94). Quetiapine can also cause significant sedation because of its binding of histamine-1 receptors as well as to alpha-1 adrenergic receptors and M1-cholinergic receptors (Figures 2-70, 2-71, and 2-94). However, the binding of H1 receptors may also enhance its ability to treat insomnia, which can be beneficial in treating not only psychosis and mania but also the depressed phase of bipolar disorder and for off-label uses such as difficult-to-treat cases of unipolar depression, various anxiety disorders, and sleep disorders.

Quetiapine can increase fasting triglyceride levels and insulin resistance, particularly at moderate to high doses, and with intermediate to high risk compared to other atypical antipsychotics (Table 2-3), possibly via the same unknown pharmacological mechanism postulated to be active for some other atypical antipsychotics (receptor X in Figures 2-58, 2-62, 2-63, 2-66, 2-67, and 2-94). Like all atypical antipsychotics, quetiapine

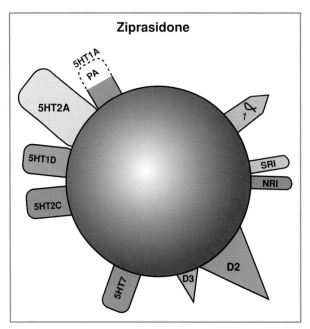

FIGURE 2-95 Ziprasidone. Ziprasidone's pharmacological icon, portraying a qualitative consensus of current thinking about the binding properties of this drug. It is the only atypical antipsychotic with serotonin (5HT) 1D antagonist and both serotonin and norepinephrine reuptake blocking properties. As with all atypical antipsychotics discussed in this chapter, binding properties vary greatly with technique and from one laboratory to another; they are constantly being revised and updated. The 5HT1A partial agonist actions as well as the 5HT2C antagonist actions may contribute to the mood-improving properties and to the cognitive enhancement observed with ziprasidone. This compound seems to lack the pharmacological actions associated with weight gain and increased cardiometabolic risk such as increasing fasting plasma triglyceride levels or increasing insulin resistance. Ziprasidone also lacks many of the pharmacological properties associated with significant sedation.

can be associated rarely with sudden and life-threatening hyperglycemic hyperosmolar syndrome/diabetic ketoacidosis; M3-cholinergic antagonism might be a factor in this, but the importance of this mechanism is still unproven (Figures 2-58, 2-64, 2-65, 2-66, 2-67, and 2-94). Actual risks versus benefits for quetiapine must be determined – as for all atypical antipsychotics – patient by patient while monitoring both efficacy and side effects, including cardiometabolic risks.

Ziprasidone. Ziprasidone has a novel chemical structure and a quite novel pharmacological profile compared to the other atypical antipsychotics (Figure 2-95). It is an SDA and is atypical in that it is associated with a low incidence of EPS and prolactin elevation. Numerous studies demonstrate that ziprasidone is highly effective for positive symptoms of schizophrenia and also improves negative symptoms of schizophrenia and the symptoms of mania in bipolar disorder. It has an intramuscular dosage formulation for rapid use in urgent circumstances that is robustly and predictably effective in acute psychosis. This is interesting, since it proves the point that ziprasidone has robust and consistent efficacy when dosed correctly, something that is not always done when ziprasidone is administered orally. When underdosed, ziprasidone, like all antipsychotics, may not exhibit full efficacy. It is now appreciated that rapid oral dose escalation to the middle or top of the dose range, while being administered twice daily with food to assure its absorption, is what provides predictability to ziprasidone's efficacy in psychosis and mania. Low doses, particularly when they are not administered with food, probably occupy too few D2 receptors for consistent efficacy. As discussed above for quetiapine, it is possible that once-daily administration of ziprasidone could be appropriate for some patients, especially if ziprasidone is taken reliably with a small (500-calorie) meal, but this has not been adequately studied.

Earlier concerns about dangerous QTc prolongation by ziprasidone now appear to be unjustified. Unlike zotepine, sertindole, and amisulpride, ziprasidone does not cause dose-dependent QTc prolongation, and few drugs have the potential to increase ziprasidone's plasma levels. Paliperidone (and by association, risperidone) also have warnings of a modest increase in QTc interval. All of these agents should be given cautiously if at all to patients receiving other drugs known to prolong QTc interval, but routine EKGs are generally not recommended. It is obviously prudent to be cautious when using any atypical antipsychotic or psychotropic drug in patients with cardiac problems or in patients taking other drugs that affect cardiac function; this is part of the routine risk-benefit calculation made for each individual patient prior to prescribing any of the atypical antipsychotic drugs.

The major differentiating feature of ziprasidone is that it has little or no propensity to promote weight gain (Table 2-2), perhaps because it has no antihistamine properties, although it does have 5HT2C-antagonist actions (Figures 2-59 and 2-95). Furthermore, there seems to be little association of ziprasidone with dyslipidemia, elevation of fasting triglycerides, or insulin resistance (Tables 2-3 and 2-4). In fact, when patients who have developed weight gain and dyslipidemia from high-risk antipsychotics (Table 2-3) are switched from those antipsychotics to ziprasidone, there can be weight loss and often lowering of fasting triglycerides while continuing to receive treatment with ziprasidone.

Is it clinically meaningful when one antipsychotic elevates cardiometabolic risk (Table 2-3) and another does not (Table 2-4)? An answer to this question can be found by considering how many patients a psychopharmacologist would have to treat with an agent that elevates cardiometabolic risk to cause one of them to get diabetes or have a heart attack (myocardial infarction), known as the number needed to harm. Progress along the metabolic highway from no disease to diabetes or myocardial infarction takes about 10 years (Figure 2-60), with loss of about 25 years of life expectancy in patients with serious mental illnesses. Statistics from clinical trials suggest that psychopharmacologists who treat patients with antipsychotics for 10 years would need to treat only about 25 male patients with olanzapine or 100 male patients with either risperidone or quetiapine to cause one of them to become diabetic in that period of time due to use of the atypical antipsychotic drug, whereas this might be predicted not to happen in anyone treated with ziprasidone (Table 2-3). Aripiprazole may also not cause increased risk of diabetes; this may also prove to be true for bifeprunox and for amisulpride, but further investigation of the latter drugs is needed (Table 2-4).

Similarly, over a 10-year period of treatment, it might require that olanzapine be administered to about 200 patients, quetiapine to 300 patients, and risperidone to 1500 patients to cause one patient to have a myocardial infarction due to the antipsychotic drug treatment, with relatively no additional risk with agents such as ziprasidone or aripiprazole. Thus, over a career of several decades, choice of atypical antipsychotic drug can make a big difference to many patients in each psychopharmacologist's practice. Sometimes incremental risks are justified by the severity of the psychotic illness, but only with metabolic monitoring can a psychopharmacologist be in a position to weigh that risk against the benefit of clinical efficacy.

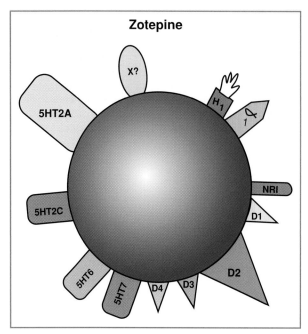

Zotepine

FIGURE 2-96 Zotepine. Zotepine's pharmacological icon, portraying a qualitative consensus of current thinking about the binding properties of this drug. As with all atypical antipsychotics discussed in this chapter, binding properties vary greatly with technique and from one laboratory to another; they are constantly being revised and updated. 5HT2C and histamine H1-antagonist properties can contribute to weight gain, H1 and alpha-1 adrenergic antagonist properties can contribute to sedation, and 5HT2C and norepinephrine reuptake inhibition (NRI) suggest possible efficacy for mood symptoms.

The pharmacological properties that make ziprasidone different in terms of its lower cardiometabolic risk are unknown but could be explained if ziprasidone lacks the ability to bind to receptors postulated to mediate insulin resistance and hypertriglyceridemia. Furthermore, ziprasidone does not bind to M3-cholinergic receptors.

Ziprasidone is the only atypical antipsychotic with 5HT1D antagonist actions as well as moderate inhibition of both 5HT reuptake and NE reuptake (Figure 2-95). These latter pharmacological actions would be expected to be both proserotonergic and pronoradrenergic, which might contribute to ziprasidone's favorable actions with regard to weight but would also predict antidepressant and anxiolytic actions. In addition, potent 5HT1A partial agonist and 5HT2C antagonist actions (Figure 2-95) may explain not only potential cognitive and affective actions of ziprasidone – due to theoretical increases in dopamine and norepinephrine in prefrontal cortex – but also the activating actions of this agent when given in subtherapeutic doses. Paradoxically, ziprasidone's activating actions may be diminished by increasing its dose. Antidepressant actions of ziprasidone are being actively tested.

Zotepine. Zotepine is an SDA available in several countries, including Japan and in Europe, has a chemical structure related to that of clozapine, but with distinguishing pharmacological (Figure 2-96) and clinical properties. Although zotepine is an SDA, some EPS have nevertheless been observed, as have prolactin elevations. Like clozapine, there is an increased risk of seizures, especially at high doses, as well as weight gain and sedation. Zotepine probably increases risk for insulin resistance, dyslipidemia, and diabetes, but it has not been extensively studied for these side effects. Unlike the case for clozapine, however, there is no clear evidence yet that zotepine is as effective for patients who fail to respond to conventional antipsychotics. Zotepine dose-dependently prolongs the QTc interval. It is generally administered three times daily. Zotepine inhibits norepinephrine reuptake

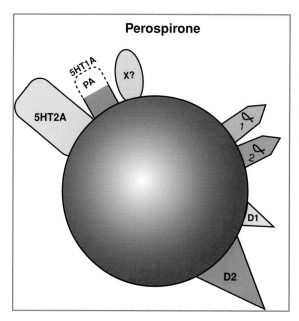

FIGURE 2-97 Perospirone. Perospirone's pharmacological icon, portraying a qualitative consensus of current thinking about the binding properties of this drug. As with all atypical antipsychotics discussed in this chapter, binding properties vary greatly with technique and from one laboratory to another; they are constantly being revised and updated. 5HT1A partial agonist actions may contribute to efficacy for mood and cognitive symptoms.

(Figure 2-96), suggesting potential antidepressant actions. Because of its side effects, zotepine is generally considered a second-line agent.

Perospirone. Perospirone is an SDA available in Japan. Its 5HT1A partial agonist actions may contribute to its efficacy (Figure 2-97). Its ability to cause weight gain, dyslipidemia, insulin resistance, and diabetes has not been well investigated. It is generally administered three times a day, and there is more experience with its use in the treatment of schizophrenia than in that of mania.

Sertindole. Sertindole is an atypical antipsychotic with SDA properties (Figure 2-98). It was originally approved in some European countries, then withdrawn for further testing of its cardiac safety and QTc-prolonging potential, and finally reintroduced into certain countries as a second-line agent. It may be useful for some patients in whom other antipsychotics have failed and who can have close monitoring of their cardiac status and drug interactions.

Loxapine. Loxapine is another SDA with a structural formula related to that of clozapine but generally classified as a conventional antipsychotic (Figure 2-99). As usually dosed, it indeed has the clinical profile of a conventional antipsychotic, causing EPS and prolactin elevation. There are hints, however, that it may be somewhat atypical at doses lower than those usually administered, and this is confirmed by human PET scans confirming its ability to block serotonin 2A receptors (see red circle in Figure 2-99) as well as D2 receptors. It is possible that loxapine's atypical properties were masked because it was used in high doses, just as high-dose use can convert other atypical antipsychotics into drugs with EPS and prolactin elevation. Testing at low doses (perhaps one-tenth of those usually administered) could confirm whether loxapine has atypical clinical properties.

Loxapine is available for intramuscular administration and usually causes no weight gain, but its cardiometabolic risk is not well characterized. A principal metabolite is N-methyl loxapine, a tricyclic antidepressant better known as amoxapine. Amoxapine has noradrenergic reuptake blocking properties, suggesting possible antidepressant actions for loxapine as well.

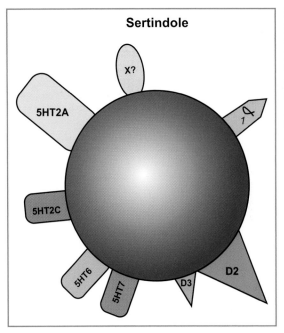

Sertindole

FIGURE 2-98 Sertindole. Sertindole's pharmacological icon, portraying a qualitative consensus of current thinking about the binding properties of this drug. As with all atypical antipsychotics discussed in this chapter, binding properties vary greatly with technique and from one laboratory to another; they are constantly being revised and updated. Potent antagonist actions at alpha-1 receptors may account for some of sertindole's side effects.

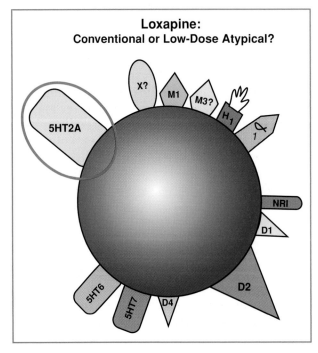

Loxapine:
Conventional or Low-Dose Atypical?

FIGURE 2-99 Loxapine. Loxapine's pharmacological icon, portraying a qualitative consensus of current thinking about the binding properties of this drug. As usually dosed, loxapine has a profile more consistent with a conventional antipsychotic than an atypical antipsychotic. However, it may be somewhat atypical at lower doses. As with all atypical antipsychotics discussed in this chapter, binding properties vary greatly with technique and from one laboratory to another; they are constantly being revised and updated. This so-called conventional antipsychotic nevertheless has antagonist actions at 5HT2A receptors (red circle), just like atypical antipsychotics, and may thus have some atypical antipsychotic properties, particularly at low doses. It also has norepinephrine reuptake inhibition (NRI) properties and has amoxapine, a known antidepressant, as one of its active metabolites; it may therefore have additional actions for mood symptoms.

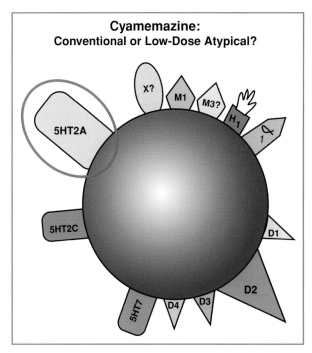

Cyamemazine: Conventional or Low-Dose Atypical?

FIGURE 2-100 Cyamemazine. Cyamemazine's pharmacological icon, portraying a qualitative consensus of current thinking about the binding properties of this drug. Like loxapine, cyemamazine's profile may be more that of a conventional antipsychotic when used at higher doses. As with all atypical antipsychotics discussed in this chapter, binding properties vary greatly with technique and from one laboratory to another; they are constantly being revised and updated. This so-called conventional antipsychotic nevertheless has antagonist actions at 5HT2A receptors (red circle) and may thus have some atypical antipsychotic properties, particularly at low doses.

Cyamemazine. Cyamemazine is another antipsychotic originally developed at high doses as a conventional antipsychotic agent with EPS and prolactin elevations, but it was subsequently found to have 5HT2A antagonist properties (see red circle in Figure 2-100). This agent is available in some European countries and has long been popular in France at low doses, especially for treating anxiety associated with psychosis. Its ability to cause weight gain and to increase cardiometabolic risk has not been extensively investigated.

Aripiprazole. This agent is the first antipsychotic developed as a D2-receptor partial agonist (DPA), a major differentiating feature from serotonin dopamine antagonists or SDAs that are silent antagonists at D2 receptors (see Figures 2-45 and 2-101). Aripiprazole does have the 5HT2A antagonist properties associated with SDAs but not the full antagonist actions at D2 receptors associated with SDAs (Figure 2-101). Aripiprazole also has 5HT1A partial agonist properties which, together with its 5HT2A antagonist properties, may contribute to its tolerability profile and efficacy (Figure 2-101). As for all antipsychotics, the actions of aripiprazole at D3 receptors remains unclear. Aripiprazole is highly effective in treating the positive symptoms of schizophrenia and manic symptoms in mania and has shown promising results as an augmenting agent in major depressive disorder. Early clinical results in bipolar depression have been disappointing. An intramuscular dosage formulation is now available. An orally disintegrating tablet and a liquid formulation are available.

Aripiprazole lacks the pharmacological properties normally associated with sedation, namely, robust alpha-1 adrenergic, M1-muscarinic cholinergic, and H1-histamine antagonist properties and thus is not generally sedating (Figure 2-101). In fact, aripiprazole can be activating in some patients, causing mild agitation or akathisia, which diminishes over time or is often decreased by dose reduction or by administering an anticholinergic agent or a benzodiazepine. In some people, therefore, the partial agonist properties might be too

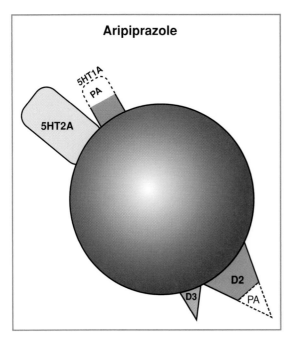

Aripiprazole

FIGURE 2-101 **Aripiprazole.** Aripiprazole's pharmacological icon, portraying a qualitative consensus of current thinking about the binding properties of this drug. Aripiprazole differs from most other antipsychotics in that it is a partial agonist at D2 receptors rather than an antagonist. As with all atypical antipsychotics discussed in this chapter, binding properties vary greatly with technique and from one laboratory to another; they are constantly being revised and updated. Additional important pharmacological properties that may contribute to its clinical profile include 5HT2A antagonist actions and 5HT1A partial agonist actions. Aripiprazole lacks the pharmacological actions usually associated with significant sedation and also seems to lack the pharmacologic actions associated with weight gain and increased cardiometabolic risk, such as increasing fasting plasma triglyceride levels or increasing insulin resistance.

close to full antagonism, with mild EPS such as akathisia (Figure 2-54), at least on dosage initiation and in patients without prior exposure to D2 full antagonists.

In other patients, the partial agonist properties might be too close to those of a dopamine agonist (Figure 2-54), with activation, nausea, and occasionally vomiting. In these cases, the use of time, dose adjustment, and short-term concomitant benzodiazepines can smooth the transition to a DPA and optimize tolerability.

A major differentiating feature of aripiprazole is that it has, like ziprasidone, little or no propensity to promote weight gain (Table 2-2), perhaps because it has no antihistamine properties or 5HT2C antagonist actions (Figures 2-59 and 2-101). Furthermore, there seems to be little association of aripiprazole with dyslipidemia, elevation of fasting triglycerides, or insulin resistance (Tables 2-3 and 2-4). In fact, as in the case of ziprasidone, when patients with weight gain and dyslipidemia caused by other antipsychotics switch to aripiprazole, there can be weight loss and a lowering of fasting triglyceride levels. The pharmacological properties that make aripiprazole different in terms of its lower metabolic risk are unknown but could be explained if aripiprazole lacks the ability to bind to postulated receptors that mediate insulin resistance and hypertriglyceridemia.

Amisulpride. Amisulpride was developed in Europe and other countries prior to full appreciation of the concept of dopamine partial agonism (DPA) (Figure 2-102). Thus it has not been tested in the same systems as newer agents, but there are some clinical hints that amisulpride is not only an atypical antipsychotic but that it has these clinical properties because it is a DPA at D2 receptors. Amisulpride has no appreciable affinity for 5HT2A or 5HT1A receptors to explain its low propensity for EPS and the observation of improvement of negative symptoms in schizophrenia, particularly at low doses. As in the case of all antipsychotics, it is not known how amisulpride's actions at D3 receptors may contribute to its clinical profile.

Amisulpride's ability to cause weight gain, dyslipidemia, and diabetes has not been extensively investigated. It may cause dose-dependent QTc prolongation. Since amisulpride

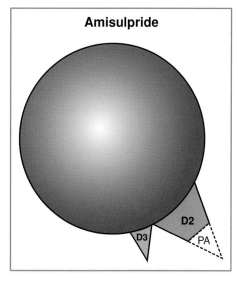

Amisulpride

FIGURE 2-102 Amisulpride. Amisulpride's pharmacological icon, portraying a qualitative consensus of current thinking about the binding properties of this drug. Amisulpride does not have affinity for serotonin 2A or 1A receptors, but it may be a partial agonist at D2 receptors rather than an antagonist. As with all atypical antipsychotics discussed in this chapter, binding properties vary greatly with technique and from one laboratory to another; they are constantly being revised and updated.

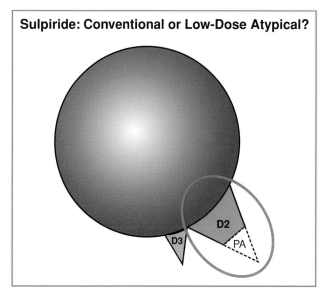

Sulpiride: Conventional or Low-Dose Atypical?

FIGURE 2-103 Sulpiride. Sulpiride's pharmacological icon, portraying a qualitative consensus of current thinking about the binding properties of this drug. At usual doses, sulpiride has the profile of a conventional antipsychotic, but at low doses it may be a partial agonist at D2 receptors, though likely still closer to the antagonist end of the spectrum. As with all atypical antipsychotics discussed in this chapter, binding properties vary greatly with technique and from one laboratory to another; they are constantly being revised and updated.

can cause prolactin elevation, if it is appropriately classifiable as a DPA, it is likely closer to a silent antagonist than is aripiprazole on the DPA spectrum and may only function as a DPA at low doses and as a more conventional D2 antagonist at high doses (see Figure 2-54).

Sulpiride. Sulpiride is an earlier compound structurally related to amisulpride that was developed as a conventional antipsychotic (Figure 2-103). Although it generally causes EPS and prolactin elevation at usual antipsychotic doses, it may be activating and have efficacy for negative symptoms of schizophrenia as well as for depression at low doses. This agent, if a DPA, is likely to have pharmacological properties very close to those of a silent antagonist and may function as a DPA only at low doses and as a more conventional D2 antagonist at high doses (Figure 2-54).

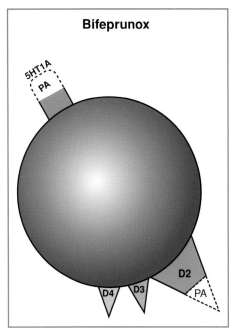

Bifeprunox

FIGURE 2-104 Bifeprunox. Bifeprunox's pharmacological icon, portraying a qualitative consensus of current thinking about the binding properties of this drug. Bifeprunox does not have appreciable affinity for serotonin 2A receptors, but instead seems to be a partial agonist at both D2 receptors and serotonin 1A receptors. As with all atypical antipsychotics discussed in this chapter, binding properties vary greatly with technique and from one laboratory to another; they are constantly being revised and updated. Bifeprunox seems to lack the pharmacological properties associated with sedation and may lack the actions that cause weight gain, or increases in fasting plasma triglycerides, or insulin resistance.

Bifeprunox.   A new DPA with efficacy for positive symptoms in schizophrenia and for manic symptoms in bipolar disorder is bifeprunox (Figure 2-104). This agent is interesting in that it has no significant 5HT2A antagonist properties but couples its DPA actions with potent 5HT1A serotonin partial agonist (SPA) actions to attain its atypical clinical profile of low EPS and a low incidence of hyperprolactinemia (Figure 2-104). Bifeprunox lacks the pharmacological properties normally associated with sedation, namely, alpha-1 adrenergic, M1-muscarinic cholinergic and H1-histamine antagonist properties; thus it is not sedating (Figure 2-104). In fact, bifeprunox can be a bit more activating than the DPA aripiprazole, thus moving it along the spectrum closer to a full agonist than aripiprazole (Figure 2-54). As a partial agonist closer to agonist actions than aripiprazole, it may cause more nausea and vomiting than aripiprazole. This can slow down the ideal rate of dose titration and thus delay onset of action in situations of acute psychosis or acute mania. On the other hand, its partial agonist actions may lead to enhanced long term tolerability during long term maintenance by having a lack of sedating side effects plus the theoretical potential to brighten patients by improving both cognitive and affective symptoms, clinical possibilities that are currently under investigation. Bifeprunox does not appear to pose a great risk of weight gain or of increasing cardiometabolic risk such as dyslipidemia, increased insulin resistance, or elevated fasting plasma triglycerides, but it is still under investigation for these properties (Table 2-4). Bifeprunox is also under study as an antidepressant for the depressed phase of bipolar disorder. The emerging clinical profile of bifeprunox is one that may be advantageous for long-term use as a maintenance agent in schizophrenia and bipolar disorder.

Antipsychotics in clinical practice

The prescription of antipsychotics in clinical practice can be very different from studying them in clinical trials. Real patients are often more complicated, may have diagnoses that do not meet diagnostic criteria for the formally studied indications, and generally have much more comorbidity than patients studied in clinical trials. Thus, it is important for the practicing psychopharmacologist to appreciate that different atypical antipsychotics can have clinically distinctive effects in different patients in clinical practice. What this also means is that median clinical effects in clinical trials may not be the best indicator of the range of clinical responses possible for individual patients. Furthermore, optimal doses suggested from clinical trials often do not match optimal doses used in clinical practice (too high for some drugs; too low for others). Finally, although virtually all studies are head-to-head comparisons of monotherapies and/or placebo, many patients receive two antipsychotics or antipsychotics plus other psychotropic drugs in clinical practice settings. Sometimes this is rational and justified, but sometimes it is not. Here we will briefly discuss some of the issues that arise in trying to apply knowledge about the pharmacological mechanisms of action discussed so far in this chapter to the utilization of atypical antipsychotics in clinical practice.

Schizophrenia symptom pharmacies

Although it is important to make accurate psychiatric diagnoses, throughout this book it has been emphasized that in reality, clinicians treat symptoms, not diseases. Psychiatric disorders are clusters of symptoms for which the underlying disease is not known, but psychopharmacological agents can be powerful agents to relieve suffering by reducing symptoms. Here we break down the syndrome of schizophrenia and psychotic illnesses into symptom dimensions in order to customize the application of treatments to specific symptoms.

Positive symptom pharmacy (Figure 2-105). The most robust action of any antipsychotic is generally its ability to reduce the positive symptoms of psychosis, such as delusions and hallucinations, and these are the symptoms often targeted first in the treatment of schizophrenia. It is very difficult to consider treatment for other symptoms until the positive symptoms are somewhat under control. When the situation is urgent, rapid delivery with a short-acting intramuscular injection may be required, and this formulation is available for several atypical and conventional antipsychotics (Figure 2-105, in case of emergency). Positive symptoms can also be treated in urgent situations for the short term with an injectable benzodiazepine.

First-line treatment of positive symptoms includes any atypical antipsychotic, either a serotonin dopamine antagonist (SDA) or a dopamine partial agonist (DPA). For non-compliant patients, positive symptoms can be managed with a depot, for which one atypical antipsychotic (the SDA risperidone) as well as several conventional antipsychotics are available. Second-line treatment of positive symptoms that have not been controlled with adequate trials of a first-line SDA or DPA would include either clozapine or a conventional antipsychotic. If all else fails, either heroic doses of one of the first- or second-line agents might be considered, a combination (combo) such as augmentation of a first-line treatment with a mood stabilizer, or polypharmacy of two antipsychotics, particularly one atypical antipsychotic with one conventional antipsychotic.

Aggressive symptom pharmacy (Figure 2-106). Patients with schizophrenia can be hostile and aggressive, toward self, staff, family, and property. This may take the form of suicide attempts, self-mutilation, poor impulse control, drug abuse, verbal abuse, physical abuse, or threatening behavior and may not directly correlate with positive symptoms. It can be a particularly difficult problem among patients in a forensic setting. Such problems are also common symptom dimensions in many psychiatric disorders other than schizophrenia, including many childhood and adolescent disorders such as conduct disorder, oppositional

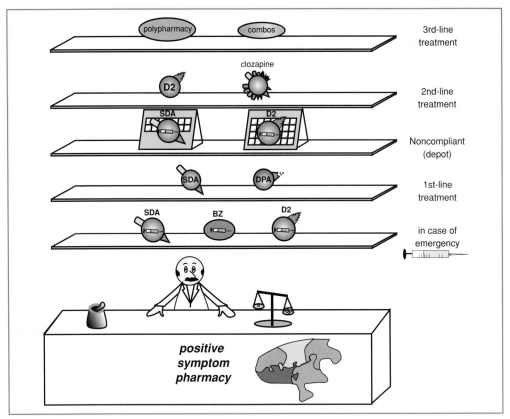

FIGURE 2-105 Positive symptom pharmacy. First-line treatment of positive symptoms is now atypical antipsychotics [serotonin-dopamine antagonists (SDAs) or dopamine partial agonists (DPAs)], not only for schizophrenia but also for positive symptoms associated with bipolar disorder, Alzheimer's disease, childhood psychoses, and other psychotic disorders. Several atypical antipsychotics are available in intramuscular formulations, which can be used acutely (in case of emergency). Conventional antipsychotics (D2) and benzodiazepines (BZ) can also be useful for acute intramuscular administration (in case of emergency). Depot injections are available for one atypical antipsychotic, risperidone (every 2 weeks) or for several conventional antipsychotics (monthly). This can be especially useful for noncompliant patients as well as for second-line use after several atypical agents fail. Clozapine, conventional antipsychotics, polypharmacy, and combinations (combos) are relegated to second- and third-line treatment for positive symptoms of psychosis.

defiant disorder, autism, mental retardation, attention deficit hyperactivity disorder, as well as borderline personality disorder, bipolar disorders, and various types of organic disorders and brain damage including head injury, traumatic brain injury, stroke, and Alzheimer's disease. This dimension of psychopathology obviously cuts a wide swath across psychiatric disorders and is not necessarily associated with psychosis.

Both conventional and atypical antipsychotics may reduce such symptoms, but there are far more studies of hostility and aggression in psychotic illnesses than in nonpsychotic illnesses. The treatment of aggressive symptoms in schizophrenia can be much like the treatment of positive symptoms with injectable antipsychotics and benzodiazepines for urgent situations, with SDA or DPA atypical antipsychotics preferred for first-line treatment (Figure 2-106). Not only clozapine or conventional antipsychotics can be helpful for aggressive symptoms in some patients when first-line treatments are not satisfactory but also oral benzodiazepines or mood stabilizers (Figure 2-106). The treatment of

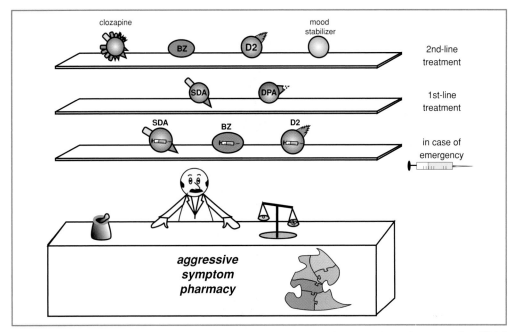

FIGURE 2-106 Aggressive symptom pharmacy. Atypical antipsychotics [serotonin-dopamine antagonists (SDAs) or dopamine partial agonists (DPAs)] are preferable (first-line) to conventional antipsychotics (D2) for the management of aggression, hostility, and impulse control because of their more favorable side effect profiles. In an acute situation, intramuscular atypical (SDA) or conventional (D2) antipsychotics as well as intramuscular benzodiazepines (BZ) may be useful. Conventional antipsychotics, clozapine, benzodiazepines, or mood stabilizers may be required when atypical antipsychotics are not effective (second-line).

hostility, aggression, and poor impulse control is always controversial; it requires good clinical judgment and consideration of other interventions such as seclusion, restraint, and environmental and milieu techniques, with prevention of utilizing drugs as punishment or excessive behavioral control vehicles ("chemical straight jackets").

The treatment of aggressive symptoms is particularly controversial when the patient does not have schizophrenia, and antipsychotics are not approved for such uses, although it may be necessary to use antipsychotics off-label for these symptoms in some cases. As mentioned earlier in this chapter, one antipsychotic, risperidone, has proven to be effective for irritability associated with autistic disorder in children and adolescents (ages 5 to 16), including symptoms of aggression toward others, deliberate self-injury, tantrums, and quickly changing moods. Although frequently used to help reduce aggression and related behavioral disturbances in dementia as well, this use must be carefully weighed against the other available options and against the risks of treatment versus the risks of nontreatment.

Negative symptom pharmacy (Figure 2-107). This symptom dimension is thought to be a particularly unique feature of schizophrenia, although certain aspects of these symptoms can overlap with symptoms that are not unique to schizophrenia itself, such as cognitive and affective symptoms. Any improvement in negative symptoms that can be gained from treatment with atypical antipsychotics is very important, because the long-term outcome of schizophrenia is more closely correlated with severity of negative symptoms than it is with that of positive symptoms. However, it is already clear that significantly more robust treatment effects will be necessary than those offered by any currently available

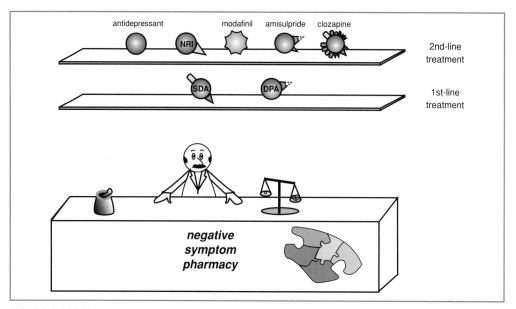

FIGURE 2-107 Negative symptom pharmacy. Negative symptoms can be improved in schizophrenia, both by switching from conventional antipsychotics (which can make these symptoms worse) to atypical antipsychotics [serotonin-dopamine antagonists (SDAs) or dopamine partial agonists (DPAs)] that do not generally worsen negative symptoms and may even improve negative symptoms. As second-line options, amisulpride or clozapine may be beneficial, as may augmentation with antidepressants, norepinephrine reuptake inhibitors (NRIs), or modafinil.

antipsychotic if such symptoms are to improve enough to transform the poor outcomes of many schizophrenic patients.

In the meantime, there are some approaches which are currently available for improving negative symptoms in the short run. First, negative symptoms secondary to antipsychotics can be readily reduced by avoiding conventional antipsychotics and by avoiding high doses of atypical antipsychotics whenever possible. Second, atypical antipsychotics actually improve negative symptoms in some patients, so first-line treatment is with either an SDA or a DPA (Figure 2-107). Finally, off-label use of certain antidepressants or cognitive enhancers can be considered as augmentation to an atypical antipsychotic. This may be helpful in selected cases.

Cognitive symptom pharmacy (Figure 2-108). Severity of cognitive symptoms correlates with the long-term prognosis of schizophrenia, so reduction of these symptoms is a vital treatment goal. The pharmacy for cognitive treatment of schizophrenia includes atypical but not conventional antipsychotics. Otherwise the cupboard is relatively bare. Augmentation with antidepressants or cognitive enhancers may be helpful in selected cases, just as these agents are occasionally helpful for negative symptoms. Discontinuing drugs with sedating or anticholinergic properties may also be useful in improving cognition in some cases. However, it is hoped that the multiple experimental interventions currently under study will be able to treat the cognitive symptoms of schizophrenia much more effectively than any of the interventions currently available, probably by adding treatments with new mechanisms to atypical antipsychotics. Many therapeutics in testing as future cognitive treatments for schizophrenia are discussed next in the final section of this chapter.

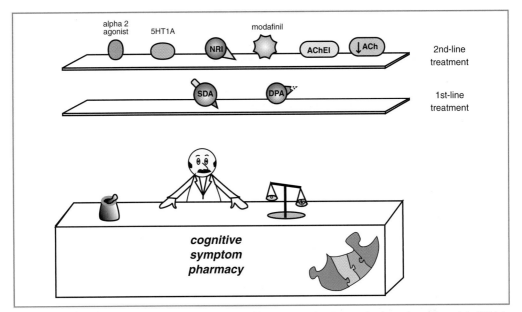

FIGURE 2-108 Cognitive symptom pharmacy. Atypical antipsychotics [serotonin-dopamine antagonists (SDAs) or dopamine partial agonists (DPAs)] may improve cognitive functions in schizophrenic patients (first-line). It may also be useful to discontinue any anticholinergic medications that you can, a welcome bonus when switching from conventional antipsychotics to atypical antipsychotics (decreased ACh). Augmentation with alpha-2 agonists, 5HT1A agonists, norepinephrine reuptake inhibitors (NRIs), modafinil, or acetylcholinesterase inhibitors (AChEIs) may all be second-line options for treating cognitive symptoms of psychosis.

Affective symptom pharmacy (Figure 2-109). Affective symptoms are a dimension of schizophrenia and are a major feature of bipolar disorder, schizoaffective disorder, and of course major depressive disorder. Further, patients with schizophrenia can even have a major depressive episode that is comorbid with their schizophrenia. Thus, it is important to treat affective symptoms in schizophrenia and bipolar disorder not only first-line with an atypical antipsychotic but also, if remission is not fully achieved with this approach, to consider augmentation with lithium, a mood stabilizer, or an antidepressant to relieve all affective symptoms and stabilize mood. Clozapine is the only atypical antipsychotic proven to reduce suicide in schizophrenia, although other antipsychotics may also be useful for this symptom. Lithium is the only mood stabilizer proven to reduce suicide in bipolar disorder, but it could possibly have a similar effect in schizophrenia, even though this has not yet been proven.

Metabolic pharmacy (Figure 2-110). Although all atypical antipsychotics approved for use in the United States are associated with metabolic warnings, experts generally believe that there are tiers of risk for weight gain (Table 2-2) as well as cardiometabolic risk among these agents (Tables 2-3 and 2-4). Thus, to avoid weight gain and cardiometabolic risk, first line treatment is either ziprasidone or aripiprazole. Monitoring is still necessary with these agents, as some patients nevertheless may exhibit weight gain or elevations in fasting triglycerides. Second-tier risk may apply to risperidone, paliperidone, and quetiapine, but monitoring is even more important among all these second tier agents (Table 2-3). Other agents that may eventually prove to belong in either the first or the second tier include bifeprunox (in testing) and amisulpride (needs further testing and available only outside the

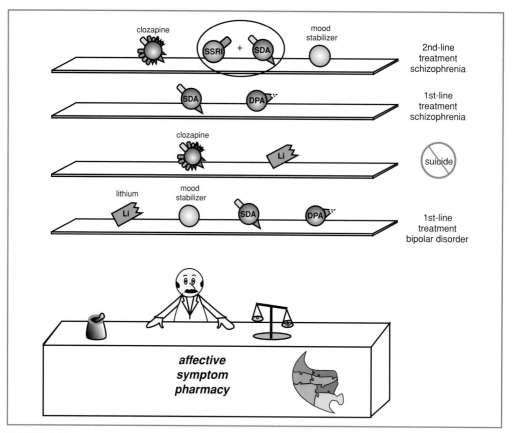

FIGURE 2-109 Affective symptom pharmacy. Atypical antipsychotics [serotonin-dopamine antagonists (SDAs) or dopamine partial agonists (DPAs)] are surprisingly effective in stabilizing mood in a number of disorders and are now becoming treatments for affective symptoms of schizophrenia (first-line), and also for stabilizing mood, mixed, rapid cycling, and treatment-resistant mood states in bipolar patients along with lithium and various anticonvulsant mood stabilizers (first-line treatment). Suicide may be reduced by clozapine (in schizophrenia) and by lithium (Li) (in bipolar disorder). Atypical antipsychotics are also combined with antidepressants such as serotonin selective reuptake inhibitors (SSRIs) or serotonin norepinephrine reuptake inhibitors (SNRIs) for affective symptoms, with clozapine or with various anticonvulsant mood stabilizers as other second-line options.

United States) (Table 2-3). The highest risk is posed by clozapine and olanzapine (Table 2-3). The actual risks of conventional antipsychotics and certain atypical antipsychotics that are available only outside the United States are not well characterized.

Sedation pharmacy (Figure 2-111). Not all antipsychotics are sedating. However, this is a side effect that can be quite variable and difficult to predict in individual patients. Those agents with the lowest risk of sedation might be aripiprazole and ziprasidone, although both can be sedating in some individuals and especially at higher doses. Bifeprunox is not often sedating. Many patients may not experience sedation with either risperidone or paliperidone, but individual experience is necessary to determine what the exact effects will be. When sedation is present with either risperidone or paliperidone, it often comes at the beginning of dosing, can return with dose escalation, and can wear off with time or be managed with once-daily nighttime administration.

In some cases, sedation may be desired. For intermittent sedation, at night or during the day, benzodiazepines are a good choice to "top up" one of the agents with a lower incidence of

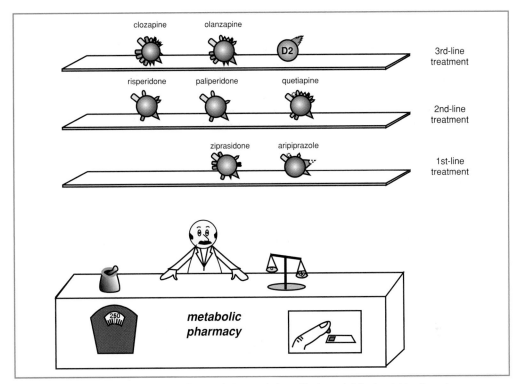

FIGURE 2-110 Metabolic pharmacy. Agents that seem to have the lowest risk of weight gain and cardiometabolic problems include ziprasidone and aripiprazole (first-line). Second-line treatment options include risperidone, paliperidone and quetiapine, while olanzapine and clozapine carry the greatest risk of weight gain and cardiometabolic effects. The risks associated with the various conventional antipsychotics (D2) are not well characterized but may be lower than the highest risk atypical antipsychotics.

sedation. However, if sedation is necessary because of incessant daytime agitation, persistent insomnia, or lack of control, patients may benefit from the artful production of sedation with appropriate doses of either quetiapine, clozapine, or olanzapine, including either daytime administration in some cases or split doses with some medication given during the day and some at night.

The art of switching antipsychotics

It might seem that it would be easy to switch from one antipsychotic to another, but this has proven to be problematic for many patients. Switching actually requires skill to convert patients from one agent to another. Otherwise, they can develop agitation, activation, insomnia, rebound psychosis, and withdrawal effects, especially anticholinergic rebound if done too quickly or without finesse (Figure 2-112).

The sophisticated clinician realizes that the way to switch patients depends on the specific antipsychotics involved and the urgency of the clinical situation. For example, clozapine might be most likely to cause rebound psychosis if rapidly discontinued. Another observation is that switching from a sedating antipsychotic to a nonsedating antipsychotic is different than switching between two sedating antipsychotics. Furthermore, switching between two agents that block D2 receptors as antagonists can be much different than switching between a D2 receptor antagonist and a DPA. These concepts are shown in the next few figures.

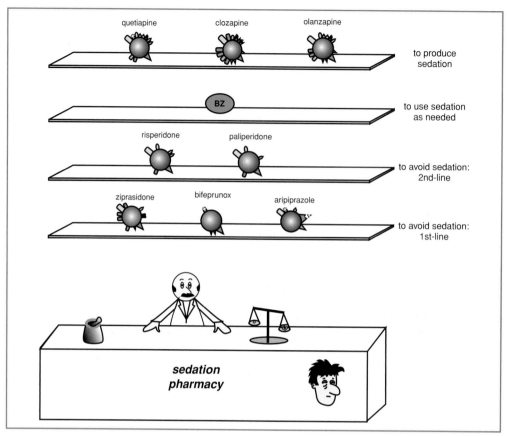

FIGURE 2-111 Sedation pharmacy. Agents that seem least likely to induce sedation include ziprasidone, aripiprazole, and bifeprunox. Risperidone and paliperidone may also not cause sedation in many patients but may cause sedation in others. In cases where sedation would be beneficial, options include quetiapine, clozapine, or olanzapine as well as augmentation with a benzodiazepine.

In general, it is rarely a good idea to precipitously stop one antipsychotic and start the other at full dose. Full doses, of course, can be given to patients who are not taking any antipsychotic at the time when one is started. However, in a switch scenario, some form of transition is usually necessary if the clinical situation is to stay stable or improve. For example, switching between two similar agents might be the easiest, such as two agents with D2 antagonist properties that are both somewhat sedating (Figure 2-113). In this case, the best results are usually obtained by cross titration over several days (Figure 2-113). This creates concomitant administration of two antipsychotics for a while as one goes up and the other goes down in dose, and this is acceptable and in fact desirable polypharmacy until the transition is complete.

Sometimes the transition between two similar agents can take up to a few weeks rather than a few days. Nevertheless, it is important to complete the transition and not get caught in cross titration, as shown in Figure 2-114. Sometimes, as the dose of the second drug goes up and the dose of the first drug comes down, the patient begins to do better, and the clinician just stops without completing the transition to a full dose of the second agent and complete discontinuation of the first. That is not generally recommended, since a full trial on the second agent is the goal, and long-term polypharmacy of two agents is not well

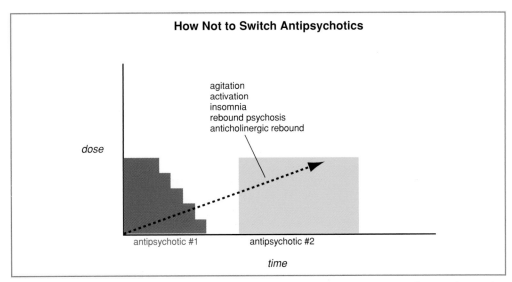

FIGURE 2-112 How not to switch antipsychotics. Converting patients from one antipsychotic to another requires great care in order to ensure that they do not develop withdrawal symptoms, rebound psychosis, or aggravation of side effects. Generally, as shown here, this means not precipitously discontinuing the first antipsychotic, allowing gaps between the administration of the two antipsychotics, or starting the second antipsychotic at full dose.

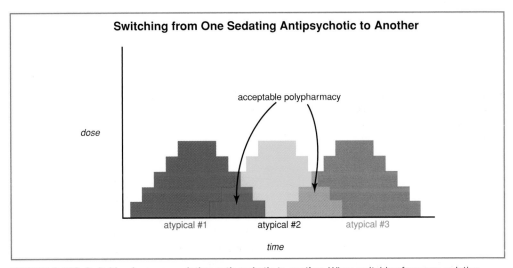

FIGURE 2-113 Switching from one sedating antipsychotic to another. When switching from one sedating antipsychotic to another, it is frequently prudent to "cross-titrate"; that is, to build down the dose of the first drug while building up the dose of the other over a few days to a few weeks. This leads to transient administration of two drugs but is justified in order to reduce side effects and the risk of rebound symptoms and to accelerate the successful transition to the second drug.

studied and can be quite expensive. If the second agent is not satisfactory, it is generally preferable to try a third rather than backtrack to the use of two agents together indefinitely (Figure 2-114).

Since the first atypical antipsychotics were all characterized as having some degree of sedation, especially at higher doses (e.g., risperidone, olanzapine, and quetiapine), it was not appreciated early that initiating treatment with a nonsedating antipsychotic (such as

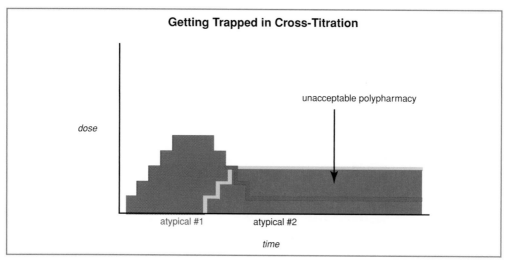

FIGURE 2-114 Getting caught in cross-titration. When switching from one atypical antipsychotic to another, the patient may improve in the middle of cross-titration. Polypharmacy results if cross-titration is stopped at this point and the patient continues both drugs indefinitely. It is generally better to complete the cross titration as shown in Figure 2-113, with discontinuation of the first agent and an adequate monotherapy trial of the second drug before trying long-term polypharmacy.

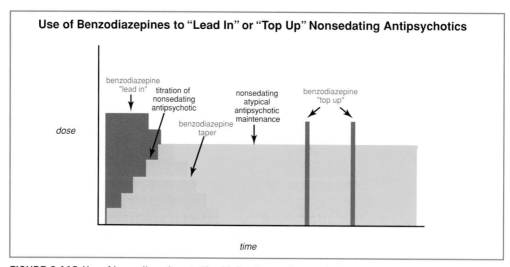

FIGURE 2-115 Use of benzodiazepines to "lead in" or "top up" nonsedating antipsychotics. Patients who are agitated and cannot sleep may need short-term augmentation with a benzodiazepine when initiating a nonsedating antipsychotic. The benzodiazepine can be discontinued once the patient is stabilized, with the potential to occasionally top up as needed.

ziprasidone or aripiprazole, introduced later to the market) and switching from a sedating to a nonsedating antipsychotic can be different. Experience now tells us that patients who are agitated and cannot sleep might need short-term supplementation with a benzodiazepine when treatment with a nonsedating agent such as aripiprazole, ziprasidone, or bifeprunox is being initiated (Figure 2-115). The disadvantage of this approach is the need to use a second drug, especially when the antipsychotic is initiated or given as a "top up" during dose stabilization. The advantage of this approach is the ability to control sedation and use it as

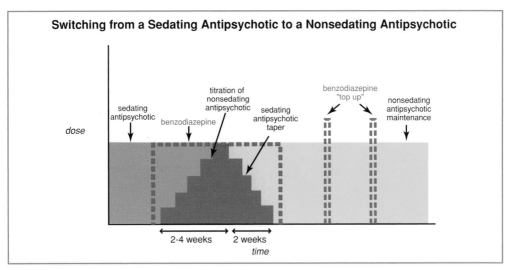

FIGURE 2-116 Switching from a sedating antipsychotic to a nonsedating antipsychotic. One method for switching from a sedating antipsychotic to a nonsedating antipsychotic shown here is to add a benzodiazepine first, and then start the up-titration of the nonsedating agent while maintaining the full dose of the sedating agent. Once the nonsedating agent is at a therapeutic dose, the sedating agent can be tapered while maintaining the benzodiazepine. Once the sedating antipsychotic is fully tapered and the patient is stable, the benzodiazepine can be tapered or stopped. In addition, once the benzodiazepine has been discontinued, it can be used as needed occasionally to top up the patient for treatment of any breakthrough agitation or insomnia. This switching method may be best for patients who are switching due to lack of adequate control of symptoms on their sedating antipsychotic rather than for those who are switching due to intolerability, as the temporary use of three agents concomitantly may cause side effects.

a therapeutic tool, discontinuing the benzodiazepine to remove unwanted sedation when it is no longer needed or desired for maintenance as well as to prevent cognitive problems and unacceptable daytime sedation once psychosis has stabilized.

Benzodiazepines can not only be useful in "leading in" and "topping up" antipsychotics when a nonsedating agent is initiated (Figure 2-115); they can also be very helpful in easing the transition from a sedating to a nonsedating antipsychotic (Figure 2-116). Thus, in preparing for a switch from a sedating agent such as quetiapine to a nonsedating agent such as aripiprazole, the switch can be anticipated by initiating a benzodiazepine before doing anything and then starting the uptitration of the nonsedating agent while maintaining the full dose of the sedating agent. This can mean the short-term use of three drugs, which can cause side effects and may not be desirable in mildly ill patients whose symptoms are under control or who are very sensitive to side effects; however, in a schizophrenic patient who is switching because of inadequate symptom control by the sedating agent, this approach, shown in Figure 2-116, should be considered, since behavioral control can be attained with the three drugs for a few days to a few weeks prior to beginning slow downtitration of the sedating antipsychotic over a few more weeks. Once the second antipsychotic has full-dose buildup and the first is completely tapered, the benzodiazepine can then be tapered and also used to top up later if necessary (Figure 2-116). This may seem complicated, but it is actually quite intuitive and allows for a successful slow transition to a nonsedating agent over several weeks without the risk of rebound psychosis or emergence of agitation and insomnia prior to giving the new agent a chance to work.

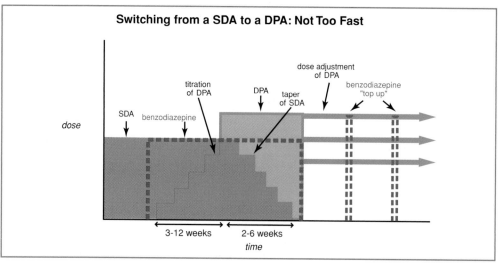

FIGURE 2-117 Switching from SDA to DPA. When switching from an agent with full D2 antagonist properties (e.g., from a serotonin-dopamine antagonist, or SDA) to a partial dopamine agonist (DPA), patients could potentially experience emergence of psychosis, agitation, or insomnia. Thus, a gradual switch may be best, with patients continuing to receive a full dose of the first antipsychotic both during uptitration of the second and perhaps for a few weeks afterward. Adding a benzodiazepine short-term may also be beneficial. Once the second antipsychotic has attained a full therapeutic dose, the first antipsychotic can be tapered while the benzodiazepine is maintained for a short time. When the patient is stable, the benzodiazepine can be discontinued, and possibly utilized again as needed occasionally to top up the patient for treatment of any breakthrough agitation or insomnia. This switch method allows the dose of the DPA to be optimized and for the dopamine receptors to potentially "reset" their sensitivity so that partial agonist actions can be optimally therapeutic.

Similar principles are at play when switching a patient from a D2 antagonist, such as an SDA, to a D2 partial agonist (DPA) (Figure 2-117). Patients accustomed to full D2 antagonism may experience less than full blockade of D2 receptors at first as they transition to a partial agonist. This can be experienced as emergence of psychosis, agitation, or insomnia but can be anticipated both by the prior initiation of a benzodiazepine and the maintenance of a full dose of the first antipsychotic for a while (Figure 2-117). It can take from a few weeks to a few months for the dopamine receptors to reset and become adequately blocked as the patient accommodates to the partial agonist and stabilizes clinically. Then, the first antipsychotic can be fully tapered, and soon thereafter the benzodiazepine as well. Dose adjustment of the DPA can be optimized once the first antipsychotic and the benzodiazepine have both been discontinued. Observing patients, anticipating and responding to their changing symptoms of psychosis and side effects during the transition, is the way to apply these tools, often utilizing time as an agent to ease the switch.

Combos and polypharmacy

Mood stabilizers can sometimes be helpful in augmenting incomplete or unsatisfactory responses of schizophrenic patients to antipsychotic monotherapy, including unsatisfactory responses to high-dose monotherapy (Figure 2-118). Lithium may not be particularly helpful in schizophrenia, but divalproex and lamotrigine or even an antidepressant can sometimes be useful as an augmenting agent to atypical antipsychotics in the treatment of schizophrenia inadequately responsive to monotherapy.

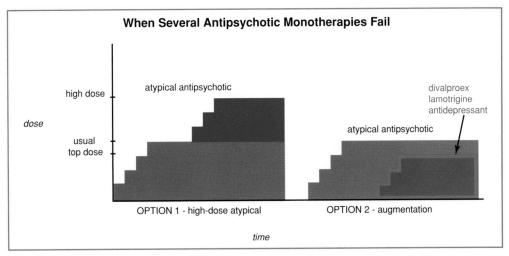

FIGURE 2-118 High dose and augmentation. When several atypical antipsychotic monotherapies fail, it may be necessary to use high doses of an antipsychotic (on the left). Although this can sometimes lead to improved efficacy, this is also quite costly and can lead to loss of the atypical therapeutic advantages of some atypical antipsychotics as well as other side effects. Another option is to add a mood stabilizer such as divalproex or lamotrigine, or an antidepressant to augment an inadequately efficacious atypical antipsychotic (on the right).

Schizophrenic patients usually respond to treatment with any single antipsychotic drug, whether conventional or atypical, by improving their positive symptoms and their total symptoms by at least 20 to 30 percent on standardized rating scales after a month or two of treatment. However, if a treatment effect of this order of magnitude is not observed after an adequate trial with the first antipsychotic agent, clinicians usually try a second, third, and fourth agent until a satisfactory response is achieved. If no satisfactory response exists to a series of monotherapies, including high doses, clozapine, and augmentation with mood stabilizers, then administration of two antipsychotics may be considered (Figure 2-119, when all else fails).

Some clinicians prefer augmenting clozapine for treatment-resistant cases, and this form of antipsychotic polypharmacy has been studied the most. Others try augmenting an atypical antipsychotic with a conventional antipsychotic or giving two atypical antipsychotics together – a very expensive proposition (Figure 2-119). Audits of antipsychotic use in clinical practice suggest that up to one-fourth of outpatients and up to half of inpatients take two antipsychotic drugs for long-term maintenance treatment. Is this a viable therapeutic option for treatment-resistant patients or a dirty little secret of irrational drug use? Whatever it is, the use of two antipsychotics seems to be one of the most practiced and least investigated phenomena in clinical psychopharmacology. It may occasionally be useful to combine two agents when no single agent is effective. On the other hand, it has not proven useful to combine two antipsychotics to get supra-additive antipsychotic effects, such as "wellness" or "awakenings." Although **depressed** patients frequently recover, **schizophrenic** patients rarely achieve wellness, no matter what drug or drug combination is given. Thus, current treatment guidelines suggest that maintenance of patients on two antipsychotics or even very high doses of atypical antipsychotics should be done sparingly and perhaps only "when all else fails" (Figure 2-119), and even in such cases only when clearly demonstrated to be beneficial.

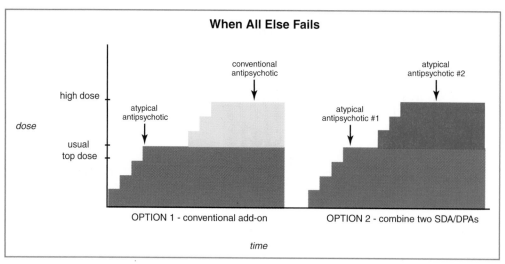

FIGURE 2-119 Polypharmacy: when all else fails. If many atypical antipsychotics show insufficient efficacy even at high doses and when augmenting agents also do not help, then a final option is to add a second antipsychotic to the first. This can be done by adding an agent from the conventional class to an atypical antipsychotic or by combining two atypical antipsychotics, whether serotonin-dopamine antagonists (SDAs) or dopamine partial agonists (DPAs). Antipsychotic polypharmacy is not well studied though frequently practiced and should truly be reserved for cases in which "all else fails."

Future treatments for schizophrenia

Innovation in the area of schizophrenia is among the most actively researched areas in psychopharmacology. New concepts of prodromal and presymptomatic treatments to prevent disease progression as well as new mechanisms aimed primarily at the devastating negative and cognitive symptoms of schizophrenia have captured the imagination of new drug discovery efforts and will be briefly reviewed here.

Presymptomatic and prodromal treatments for schizophrenia: putting the cart before the horse or preventing disease progression?

An emerging concept in psychopharmacology is the possibility that treatments that reduce symptoms could also be disease-modifying (Figure 2-120). In this chapter we have discussed how atypical antipsychotics treat symptoms of schizophrenia (first- and second-episode treatment in Figure 2-120). These same agents are also proven to prevent the reemergence of symptoms and thus relapse (maintenance treatment in Figure 2-120). It now is being debated whether these agents given to high-risk individuals either in a presymptomatic state or with only mild prodromal symptoms could prevent or delay progression to schizophrenia.

Current concepts about the natural history of schizophrenia hypothesize that this illness progresses from a state of high risk without symptoms (presymptomatic) to a prodrome with cognitive and negative but not psychotic symptoms and ultimately to a first episode with psychotic symptoms (Figure 2-120). Throughout the field of psychiatry, it is being debated whether remission of symptoms of any psychiatric disorder with psychopharmacological treatments can prevent disease progression, possibly by preventing the plastic changes in brain circuits that fully establish and worsen psychiatric disorders. In schizophrenia, therefore, the question is whether "prophylactic" antipsychotics can keep an individual from "catching" schizophrenia.

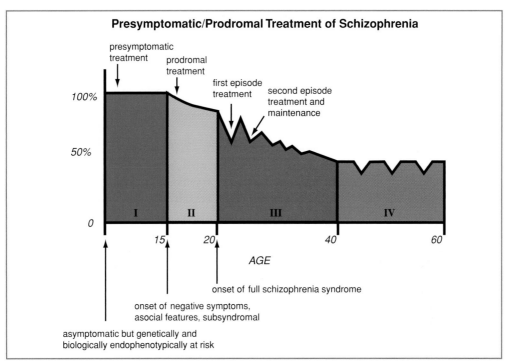

FIGURE 2-120 Presymptomatic/prodromal treatment of schizophrenia. The stages of schizophrenia are shown here over a lifetime. The patient often has full functioning (100 percent) early in life and is virtually asymptomatic (stage I). However, during a prodromal phase (stage) starting in the teens, there may be odd behaviors and subtle negative symptoms. The acute phase of the illness usually announces itself fairly dramatically in the twenties (stage), with positive symptoms, remissions, and relapses but never a complete return to previous levels of functioning. This is often a chaotic stage of the illness, with a progressive downhill course. The final phase of the illness (stage) may begin in the forties or later, with prominent negative and cognitive symptoms and some waxing and waning during its course, but often more of a burnout stage of continuing disability. There may not necessarily be a continuing and relentless downhill course, but the patient may become progressively resistant to treatment with antipsychotic medications during this stage. An emerging concept in psychopharmacology is that the treatments that reduce symptoms could also be disease modifying. That is, perhaps these agents given to high risk individuals either in a presymptomatic (stage I) or prodromal (stage 2) state could prevent or delay progression through the subsequent stages of schizophrenia.

Pilot results from early intervention studies in first-episode cases of schizophrenia already suggest that treatment with atypical antipsychotics as soon as possible after onset of the first psychotic symptoms can improve outcomes (first-episode treatment in Figure 2-120). What if high-risk patients without symptoms could be identified from genetic or neuroimaging techniques? How about patients with the prodromal cognitive and negative symptoms that frequently precede the onset of psychotic symptoms? Could treatment of patients at these points prevent the long-term course of schizophrenia – for many patients one of waxing and waning positive symptoms with ever-worsening cognitive and negative symptoms (Figure 2-120)?

Early results with atypical antipsychotics are indeed promising. Treating prodromal symptoms with antidepressants and anxiolytics may also delay the onset of schizophrenia. At this point, much more research will be required before presymptomatic or prodromal treatment can be recommended for schizophrenia, but the promise of disease-modifying treatments for psychiatric disorders in general and schizophrenia in particular is leading to studies to fully investigate this exciting possibility.

Glutamate-linked mechanisms and new treatments for schizophrenia

Much of the discussion of treatments for schizophrenia in this chapter has revolved around modifying the neurotransmitters dopamine and serotonin. A major new area of research is to investigate whether modifications of glutamate pharmacology will lead to new psychopharmacological therapeutics for schizophrenia. Targeting of the glutamate system is a logical extension of the NMDA receptor hypofunction hypothesis of schizophrenia discussed in detail in Chapter 1 and illustrated in Figures 1-39 through 1-42.

Glutamate agonists or antagonists for schizophrenia?

NMDA antagonists. Throughout this chapter, we have discussed the idea that the dopamine system should be optimized or even "stabilized" in schizophrenia, with neither too much nor too little dopamine activity in various pathways throughout the brain. A very similar concept could be applied to the glutamate system. That is, one hypothesis of schizophrenia suggests that early in the illness, excessive glutamate activity could lead to excitotoxicity (discussed in Chapter 1 and illustrated in Figures 1-45 through 1-52) and thus interfere with normal neurodevelopment (Figure 1-52). Excitotoxicity could also continue during the course of the illness and be linked to disease progression in schizophrenia (Figures 1-44 and 2-120). However, it is now also widely hypothesized that once the illness of schizophrenia has developed, NMDA glutamate receptors are actually hypofunctional (discussed in Chapter 1 and illustrated in Figures 1-39 through 1-41). So what is the best approach to treatment for schizophrenia, glutamate agonists or glutamate antagonists? The answer may be that it depends on what stage of the illness is being treated, what specific symptoms are being targeted, and whether either the agonist or antagonist action modulates the glutamate system by tuning it, stabilizing it, and optimizing it, or is too powerful and either shuts it down or overly stimulates it.

Thus, the idea has arisen that blocking excessive and excitotoxic glutamate neurotransmission (Figures 1-45 through 1-52) with NMDA antagonists might prevent damage or death to neurons in schizophrenia (Figure 2-121). It may also be possible to prevent neuronal death or damage after excessive glutamate neurotransmission by administering free radical scavengers (Figure 2-122), which destroy free radicals generated during glutamate-mediated excitotoxicity (Figures 1-49 through 1-51). Although this idea of blocking NMDA neurotransmission and its consequences has a certain theoretical appeal for the treatment of schizophrenia, especially for preventing possible neuronal damage at critical points during neurodevelopment (Figure 1-52), it may be more applicable to other conditions where excitotoxic neurodegenerative activity remains an active component of the disease mechanism, such as Alzheimer's disease and other neurodegenerative conditions. In schizophrenia, there may be a combination both of excitotoxicity, particularly early in the disease process (Figure 1-52), and NMDA receptor hypoactivation during the later course of the disease (Figures 1-39 to 1-42), making the use of agents that block NMDA receptors potentially quite complicated.

Thus potent NMDA antagonists might block excitotoxicity, but at a price: they would also cause or worsen positive, cognitive, and negative symptoms of schizophrenia (Figure 2-121). In fact, we have already discussed how the observations that NMDA antagonists such as phencyclidine (PCP) or ketamine can produce the symptoms of schizophrenia in normal volunteers is consistent with the NMDA receptor hypofunction hypothesis of schizophrenia. This seems to be too dear a price to pay for neuroprotection in schizophrenia.

One response to this quandary is to consider whether less robust NMDA antagonists such as memantine or even amantadine, that only partially block NMDA neurotransmission,

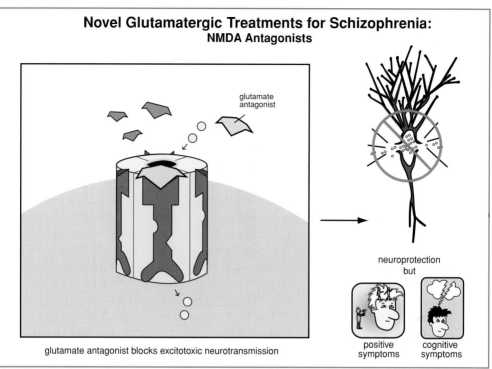

Novel Glutamatergic Treatments for Schizophrenia:
NMDA Antagonists

glutamate antagonist

glutamate antagonist blocks excitotoxic neurotransmission

neuroprotection but

positive symptoms

cognitive symptoms

FIGURE 2-121 Novel glutamatergic treatments for schizophrenia: NMDA antagonists? Antagonists of glutamate either at the N-methyl-d-aspartate (NMDA) agonist site as shown here, or at any number of allosteric sites around this receptor complex, could potentially block excitotoxic neurotransmission and exert neuroprotective actions. Such agents would potentially be treatments for conditions characterized by ongoing excitotoxic neurodegeneration such as schizophrenia, Alzheimer's disease, or other neurodegenerative conditions. Theoretically, they could also be useful for preventing early excitotoxic neuronal damage in schizophrenia. However, later in the course of schizophrenia there seems to be NMDA receptor hypoactivation that contributes to the pathophysiology of positive and cognitive symptoms. Thus, NMDA antagonists could actually worsen those symptoms.

might be better options. Another possibility is to block the presynaptic release of glutamate, which is the hypothesized mechanism of certain anticonvulsants that also act as mood stabilizers, like lamotrigine and riluzole. Blockade of presynaptic release of glutamate by agonists acting at presynaptic metabotropic glutamate receptors (mGluR2/3) is discussed below and illustrated in Figure 2-125. Much of the current targeting of the glutamate system in schizophrenia, however, is now aiming at psychopharmacological mechanisms whereby glutamate neurotransmission can actually be **increased** to compensate for NMDA receptor **hypoactivity**, but without increasing it so much as to become neurotoxic.

Glycine agonists. In Chapter 1 we discussed the actions of coagonists at the glycine site of NMDA receptors (Figures 1-34 and 1-35). Agonists at the glycine site of NMDA receptors include the naturally occurring amino acids glycine (Figure 1-34) and d-serine (Figure 1-35). An analogue of d-serine called d-cycloserine is also active at the glycine coagonist site of NMDA receptors. All of these agents have been tested in schizophrenia, with evidence that they can reduce negative and/or cognitive symptoms (Figure 2-123). Further testing is in progress, and synthetic agonists with greater potency are in

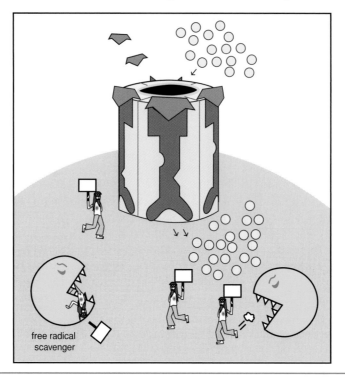

Novel Glutamatergic Treatments for Schizophrenia:
Free Radical Scavengers for Excitotoxicity

free radical
scavenger

FIGURE 2-122 Novel glutamatergic treatments for schizophrenia: free radical scavengers for excitotoxicity. Free radicals are generated in the neurodegenerative process of excitotoxicity. A drug acting as a free radical scavenger, which works as a "chemical sponge," soaking up toxic free radicals and removing them, would be theoretically neuroprotective. Vitamin E is one such weak scavenger. Other free radical scavengers, such as the lazaroids (so named because of their putative properties of raising degenerating neurons, like Lazarus, from the dead) are also being tested.

discovery. Perhaps stimulation of the glycine site will boost NMDA receptor activity enough to overcome its hypothetical hypofunction (Figures 1-39 to 1-42) and thereby reduce not only negative and cognitive symptoms, but possibly even affective symptoms in schizophrenia (Figure 2-123) without worsening positive symptoms or becoming neurotoxic.

GlyT1 inhibitors. Earlier, in Chapter 1, we also discussed how glycine transporters on glial cells, known as GlyT1, terminate the action of glycine released by glial cells into the synapses to act at the glycine site of NMDA receptors (Figure 1-34). Several GlyT1 inhibitors are now in testing, including the natural agent N-methyl-glycine, also known as sarcosine, as well as drugs in preclinical testing, such as SSR 504734, SSR 241586, JNJ17305600, and Org 25935. GlyT1 inhibitors are analogous to drugs that inhibit reuptake of other neurotransmitters, such as the serotonin selective reuptake inhibitors (SSRIs) and their actions at the serotonin transporter, or SERT. When GlyT1 pumps are blocked by a GlyT1 inhibitor, this increases the synaptic availability of glycine and thus enhances NMDA neurotransmission (Figure 2-124). Sarcosine has been shown to improve negative, cognitive, and depressive symptoms, including symptoms such as alogia and blunted affect in schizophrenia. The hope is that GlyT1 inhibitors with greater potency, such as those in preclinical testing mentioned above, will be able to reduce the hypofunctioning of NMDA

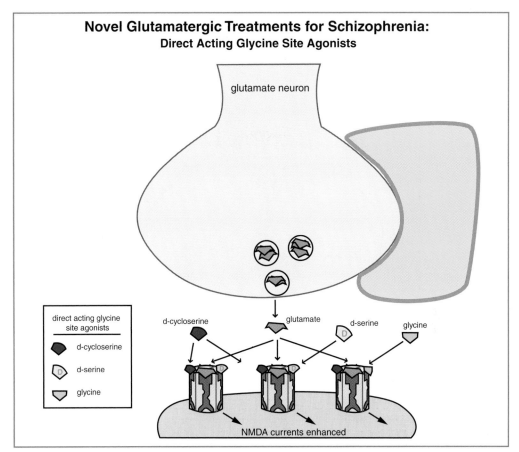

Novel Glutamatergic Treatments for Schizophrenia:
Direct Acting Glycine Site Agonists

glutamate neuron

direct acting glycine site agonists

d-cycloserine

d-serine

glycine

d-cycloserine

glutamate

d-serine

glycine

NMDA currents enhanced

FIGURE 2-123 Novel glutamatergic treatments for schizophrenia: direct acting glycine site agonists.
N-methyl-d-aspartate (NMDA) receptors require the presence of both glutamate and a coagonist at the glycine site in order to be fully active. Since schizophrenia may be linked to hypoactive NMDA receptors, agonists at the glycine coagonist site may boost glutamate neurotransmission at NMDA receptors in a manner sufficient to reduce hypoactivity and enhance NMDA currents, but not so much as to cause excitotoxicity. Several agonists at this coagonist site – including glycine, d-serine, and d-cycloserine – have been tested in schizophrenia and indeed show evidence that they can reduce negative and/or cognitive symptoms. Glycine agonists may thus be promising future treatments for negative and cognitive symptoms of schizophrenia without worsening positive symptoms.

receptors and lead to improvements particularly in the negative, cognitive, and affective symptoms of schizophrenia without activating positive symptoms or becoming neurotoxic.

mGluR2/3 presynaptic agonists. Another class of glutamate receptor, known as metabotropic glutamate receptors (mGluRs), regulates neurotransmission at glutamate synapses as well (discussed in Chapter 1 and illustrated in Figures 1-36 and listed in Table 1-11). Normally, presynaptic mGluR2/3s act as autoreceptors to prevent glutamate release (Figure 1-37B). Thus, stimulating this action with a selective presynaptic mGluR2/3 agonist could potentially stop glutamate release from the presynaptic glutamate neuron (Figure 2-125). Compounds with this action include LY404039, LY35470, LY379268 and MSG0028. The amino acid analog LY404039 is not absorbed very well after oral administration, so an inactive prodrug that is a methionine amide of this drug has been developed for human testing, known as LY2140023. LY2140023 can be absorbed orally and is then hydrolyzed to produce the active selective mGluR2/3 agonist LY404039. Thus,

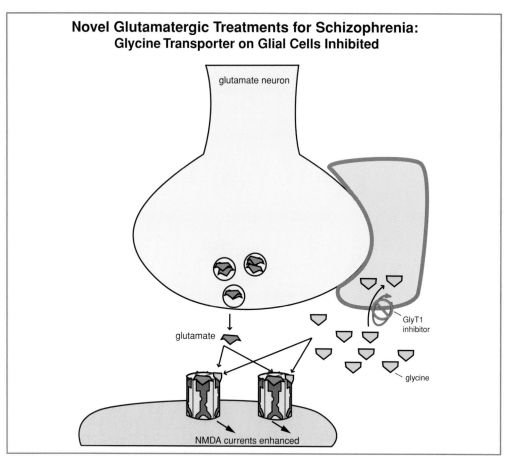

FIGURE 2-124 Novel glutamatergic treatment for schizophrenia: Glycine transporter on glial cells inhibited.
The glycine transporter-1 (GlyT1) normally terminates the actions of glycine at NMDA receptors in the glutamate synapse by transporting the glycine back up into glial cells as a reuptake pump. Thus, inhibitors at the glycine transporter-1 would increase availability of synaptic glycine, enhancing activity at NMDA receptors and enhancing NMDA currents. This is analogous to the actions of an SSRI (serotonin selective reuptake inhibitor) at serotonin synapses. GlyT1 inhibition could potentially improve cognitive and negative symptoms of schizophrenia by enhancing the availability of glycine at hypofunctioning NMDA receptors. Preclinical evidence does suggest cognitive improvements with GlyT1 inhibition, and one such naturally occurring inhibitor sarcosine has been shown to improve the negative, cognitive, and depressive symptoms of schizophrenia, including symptoms such as alogia and blunted affect.

LY2140023 has been tested in schizophrenic patients with early findings of significant improvement of positive and negative symptoms of schizophrenia compared to placebo. If confirmed, this would be the first example of an antipsychotic agent that does not directly block dopamine 2 receptors.

Why might one wish to block glutamate release in schizophrenia? One possibility is that the hypothetically hypofunctional NMDA receptors might actually lead to a compensatory increase in glutamate release in a futile attempt to overcome the malfunction at NMDA receptors. Stopping this pathological increase in glutamate release may be helpful in reducing symptoms of schizophrenia. In fact, when the NMDA antagonist PCP (phencyclidine), a drug capable of producing a human model of schizophrenia (discussed in chapter 1), is

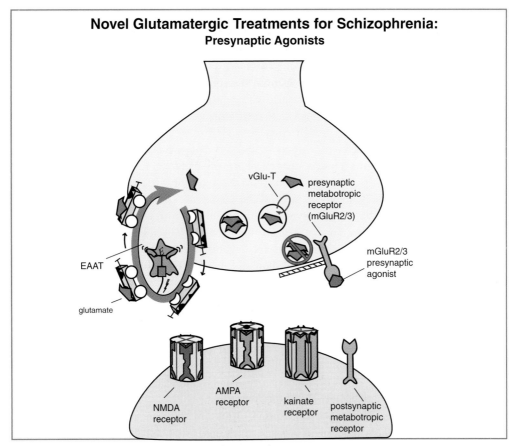

Novel Glutamatergic Treatments for Schizophrenia:
Presynaptic Agonists

vGlu-T

presynaptic
metabotropic
receptor
(mGluR2/3)

mGluR2/3
presynaptic
agonist

EAAT

glutamate

NMDA
receptor

AMPA
receptor

kainate
receptor

postsynaptic
metabotropic
receptor

FIGURE 2-125 Novel glutamatergic treatments for schizophrenia: presynaptic agonist. Presynaptic metabotropic glutamate receptors (mGluR2/3) act as autoreceptors to prevent glutamate release. Thus, stimulating these receptors could block glutamate release, and thereby decrease activity at postsynaptic glutamate receptors. Also shown is the presynaptic reuptake pump for glutamate, the excitatory amino acid transporter (EAAT) and the synaptic vesicle transporter for glutamate or vGluT. Shown postsynaptically are not only NMDA receptors, but also AMPA (alpha-amino-3-hydroxy-5-methyl-4-isoxazolepropionic acid) receptors, kainate receptors, and postsynaptic metabotropic receptors, all for glutamate.

given to experimental animals, the behavioral changes seen in these animals are reversed by selective presynaptic mGluR2/3 agonists. This is consistent with improvement of function due to reduction of glutamate release. Presynaptic agonists at mGluR2/3 receptors may also indirectly reduce dopamine neurotransmission, act as indirect 5HT2A antagonists (see Figure 2-31) and be neuroprotective. Much more research will be necessary to confirm whether mGluR2/3 agonists will become novel treatments for schizophrenia, and to clarify how they work.

AMPA-kines. AMPA receptors are another glutamate receptor subtype that regulate ion flow and neuronal depolarization that can lead to NMDA receptor activation. A number of modulators of the AMPA receptor are under development, including those that do not act directly at the glutamate site of this receptor but at positive allosteric modulating (i.e., PAM) sites on this receptor (e.g., CX 516). Sometimes these AMPA PAMs are also called AMPA-kines. Preliminary evidence from animal studies suggest that AMPA-kines might enhance cognition, but early results with CX516 in schizophrenia are disappointing. However, more potent AMPA-kines are being developed (CX546, CX619/Org 24448, Org 25573, Org 25271, Org 24292, Org 25501, and LY293558), and these might have more efficacy for cognitive symptoms in schizophrenia without showing activation of positive symptoms or neurotoxicity.

Sigma-1 agonists/antagonists. Sigma-1 receptors may be associated not only with the psychotomimetic actions of PCP but also with regulation of the NMDA receptor. However, the exact physiological functions of sigma receptors and how they may modulate NMDA receptor functioning remain poorly characterized; thus sigma-1 receptors remain in many ways the "sigma enigma."

Theoretically, sigma-1 antagonists may have actions similar to those of PCP at NMDA receptors, resulting in hypofunctioning NMDA receptors. It is possible that sigma-1–selective antagonists could block any PCP-like actions occurring in schizophrenia and thus might reverse NMDA receptor hypofunction. It might, however, cause NMDA receptor hypofunction of its own. In that case, it might be more useful to administer a sigma-1 agonist. Until there are selective agonists, antagonists, and partial agonists of the sigma-1 receptor, it will not be clear whether there is any merit to this hypothesis. Furthermore, testing of sigma receptors in schizophrenia is just beginning, especially as more selective compounds such as BMY-14802, SSR125047, and SR31742A become available. A combined sigma/5HT1A agonist/5HT reuptake inhibitor OPC14523 is being tested in depression. The SSRI fluvoxamine is not only an inhibitor of SERT, but also acts at sigma receptors, perhaps as a sigma-1 agonist, with some preclinical evidence that fluvoxamine can improve PCP-induced cognitive deficits.

Novel serotonin- and dopamine-linked mechanisms

New serotonin 2A/D2 antagonists (SDAs). Other SDAs are on the horizon and include iloperidone, an SDA with potent alpha-1 antagonist properties, whose efficacy has been primarily linked to specific pharmacogenetic markers, and whose tolerability is linked to CYP2D6 activity. Another SDA in late development is asenapine, structurally related to mirtazapine, which has potent alpha-2 antagonist properties, possibly predicting antidepressant actions, as well as potent actions on a number of 5HT receptor subtypes, possibly predicting actions for negative, affective, and cognitive symptoms in schizophrenia. Several other new SDAs are shown in Figure 2-38.

5HT2A-selective antagonists/inverse agonists. The role of 5HT2A receptors in the regulation of dopamine release was discussed earlier in this chapter and illustrated in Figures 2-21 and 2-22. Drugs with 5HT2A antagonist properties as well as D2 antagonist properties – namely, the class of SDAs – can thus balance prodopaminergic actions with antidopaminergic properties. However, to get the prodopaminergic actions inherent in the 5HT2A-antagonist mechanism may require high dosing and thus a degree of concomitant D2-antagonist action that prevents the ideal balance of dopamine release with dopamine blockade. One solution to this could be to dose the SDA agent for ideal D2 blockade (perhaps as low as 70 percent receptor blockade in mesolimbic pathways) and then to supplement the concomitant 5HT2A-receptor antagonism with a second agent that has pure 5HT2A-antagonist properties, resulting in the desired portfolio of net actions, namely complete blockade of 5HT2A receptors and incomplete but substantial blockade of D2 receptors.

Recently a 5HT2A inverse agonist, ACP 103, has entered clinical testing, with early clinical evidence that the augmentation of lower doses of antipsychotics such as risperidone may enhance efficacy in schizophrenia and possibly reduce side effects. This approach could potentially convert conventional antipsychotics into atypical antipsychotics or allow dose sparing of atypical antipsychotics, or it could optimize the efficacy and safety profile of various antipsychotics; however, further testing will be required. Earlier testing of MDL 100907 was discontinued. Another compound with this mechanism at 5HT2A receptors is eplivanserin (SR 46349).

Serotonin 1A agonists or antagonists. Theoretically, the 5HT1A actions of some atypical antipsychotics may contribute to their clinical properties, from procognitive actions to antidepressant actions to anxiolytic actions. There is debate as to whether the ideal 5HT1A actions are agonist, partial agonist, or antagonist actions, although in many cases the net long-term consequences are similar since antagonists block and chronic agonists down regulate 5HT1A receptors. Early studies with 5HT1A partial agonists such as buspirone and tandospirone added on to antipsychotics suggest possible improvement in cognition in schizophrenia. Other agents in this class include the 5HT1A partial agonist gepirone ER, the 5HT1A partial agonist/serotonin reuptake inhibitors vilazodone and Lu AA21004, and the selective 5HT1A antagonists lecozotan (SRA133) and AV965.

Serotonin 2C agonists or antagonists. Theoretically, the 5HT2C actions of some atypical antipsychotics may also contribute to their clinical actions, including procognitive and antidepressant actions. A 5HT2C agonist may be expected to reduce positive symptoms by reducing dopamine release in the mesolimbic dopamine pathway. Vabicaserin (SCA-136) is a 5HT2C agonist that has shown promise in preliminary testing in schizophrenia.

On the other hand, 5HT2C antagonists may be expected to reduce depression and improve cognition by enhancing dopamine release in the mesocortical dopamine pathway and also to release norepinephrine in the same brain areas. Several atypical antipsychotics have 5HT2C antagonist actions (see Figures 2-90 through 2-104), as does the SSRI antidepressant fluoxetine and the novel antidepressant agomelatine. The debate on whether the desired 5HT2C actions are agonist, partial agonist, or antagonist actions continues, as it does for 5HT1A receptors, although long-term actions may be similar for agents across the agonist spectrum, since antagonists block and chronic agonists may downregulate 5HT2C receptors.

5HT6 antagonists. The physiological role of 5HT6 receptors is still being clarified, but it does appear that these receptors may be linked to the production and/or release of neurotrophic factors such as brain derived neurotrophic factor (BDNF). Some atypical antipsychotics do have 5HT6-antagonist properties (clozapine, Figure 2-90; olanzapine, Figure 2-91; quetiapine, Figure 2-94; zotepine, Figure 2-96; sertindole, Figure 2-98; loxapine, Figure 2-99; and perhaps others), which might increase the release of BDNF, although it is not known whether this contributes to any of the possible protrophic effects seen with antipsychotics. Selective 5HT6-receptor antagonists such as GW742457 are in development for testing in both schizophrenia and depression and other disorders where protrophic actions on BDNF could exert a therapeutic action.

5HT7 antagonists. The physiological role of 5HT7 receptors is also being clarified, and some atypical antipsychotics do have 5HT7 actions (clozapine, Figure 2-90; risperidone, Figure 2-91; paliperidone, Figure 2-92; quetiapine, Figure 2-94; ziprasidone, Figure 2-95; zotepine, Figure 2-96; sertindole, Figure 2-98; loxapine, Figure 2-99; cyamemazine, Figure 2-100; and possibly others), even though it is not known whether this contributes to their therapeutic effects. 5HT7 receptors may be linked to circadian rhythms, sleep, anxiety and depression; selective 5HT7 antagonists are being developed and tested not only in schizophrenia but also in other psychiatric disorders such as sleep, mood, and anxiety disorders.

New DPAs. Several new dopamine partial agonists (DPAs) are in development, including bifeprunox (DU 127090), a DPA with 5HT1A partial agonist properties that is pending marketing and in late clinical development in many countries (Figure 2-53). Several compounds mix DPA actions (dopamine 2-receptor partial agonist) with SPA actions (serotonin 1A partial agonist), including sarizotan (EMD128130), SSR181507, SLV313, and SLV314. Two of these compounds are related to bifeprunox, including SLV313, which appears to balance relatively selective D2 and 5HT1A partial agonist activities, and SLV314, which is a potent DPA with serotonin reuptake inhibition properties but less potent actions at 5HT1A receptors.

Selective D3 antagonists. The function of D3 receptors remains unknown, and until recently was difficult to study since it was not possible to separate D2-antagonist properties from D3-antagonist properties of antipsychotics. Now that D3-selective agents are available, preclinical testing suggests that these agents may be useful for both negative symptoms and cognitive symptoms and might reduce stimulant abuse both in schizophrenia and in patients with substance abuse disorders who do not have schizophrenia. One example of this is RGH 188, with D3 and D2 partial agonist actions.

Other dopamine mechanisms. D1-selective agonists may be useful as procognitive agents. This may be helpful in other cognitive disorders as well. Since some atypical antipsychotics are D1 antagonists, D1-agonist action may help reverse the undesirable actions of D1 antagonism.

Many atypical antipsychotics are also D4 antagonists, and selective D4 antagonists (such as YM-43611, nemonapride, fananserin, L-745870, PNU-101387G, NGD-94–4, LU-111995, and LU35138) have been synthesized and several tested in schizophrenia, but they have not been found to be helpful.

Modafinil is an agent approved for sleepiness and may improve attention in several sleep disorders. It has also been shown to improve cognitive functioning in attention deficit hyperactivity disorder. Modafinil may act in part as a dopamine transport (DAT) inhibitor, and it as well as other DAT inhibitors could potentially improve cognition in schizophrenia and other disorders but might also activate psychosis.

Centrally acting COMT inhibitors. Catechol-O-methyl transferase inhibitors can boost the actions of dopamine, and those that act peripherally can be given with levodopa to reduce the peripheral metabolism of levodopa and enhance the central actions of dopamine. Centrally acting COMT inhibitors have the potential of increasing dopamine neurotransmission directly in the brain, especially in prefrontal cortex, where COMT is the key metabolic pathway for dopamine degradation.

Norepinephrine-linked mechanisms. Norepinephrine-selective reuptake inhibitors have been tested in depression and in attention deficit hyperactivity disorder. Norepinephrine reuptake inhibitors enhance the release not just of norepinephrine but also of dopamine in prefrontal cortex and thus may enhance executive functioning. Some preliminary investigation of this mechanism for cognitive dysfunction in schizophrenia is in progress.

Acetylcholine-linked mechanisms

Alpha-7-nicotinic cholinergic agonists. The alpha-7-nicotinic cholinergic receptor has been implicated in the familial transmission of sensory gating deficits in families with schizophrenia. Deficits in activity at this receptor could theoretically predispose patients to problems with learning efficiency and accuracy and underlie delusional thinking and social dysfunction. In addition, heavy smoking in many schizophrenics (about two-thirds of a North American population of schizophrenics are smokers; in comparison, about one-fourth of nonschizophrenics are smokers) is consistent with the high concentration of nicotine necessary to activate the receptor and with the receptor's rapid desensitization. Thus there are numerous theoretically appealing hypotheses to targeting this receptor to improve particularly cognitive functioning in schizophrenia and other cognitive disorders. Preliminary testing of DMXB-A {3-[(2,4-dimethoxy) benzylidene] anabaseine}, a natural alkaloid derivative and partial agonist at alpha-7-nicotinic cholinergic receptors, appears to have some positive effects on cognition in schizophrenia. Other alpha-7-nicotinic cholinergic agonists in testing include ABT089, MEM3454, and SSR180711.

Alpha-4 Beta-2 partial agonists (nicotinic partial agonists, or NPAs). A second subtype of nicotinic receptor may be involved in mediating the reward mechanisms of smoking – namely the alpha-4 beta-2 nicotinic acetylcholine receptor located in the mesolimbic reward pathway. Recently a number of partial agonists for this receptor have been identified, namely selective alpha-4 beta-2 nicotinic acetylcholine partial agonists, or NPAs. One of these, varenicline, has been approved for smoking cessation, and other compounds such as SSR591813 and TC1827 are in testing. Since a great number of schizophrenic patients smoke, which enhances their cardiometabolic risk and can reduce their life expectancy, already abnormal due to factors linked to their psychiatric illness, lifestyle, and some of their treatments, it seems important to investigate treatments that could reduce smoking. Most studies of varenicline have involved patients without psychiatric disorders and who do not take psychotropic drugs; testing is now needed to determine to what extent NPAs are effective in reducing smoking specifically in schizophrenic patients who take antipsychotics.

Muscarinic-1 agonists. Muscarinic-1 (M1) antagonist properties of antipsychotics contribute to sedation and cognitive dysfunction, so it seems logical to determine whether an M1 agonist would be procognitive in schizophrenia or other cognitive disorders. ACP104, a metabolite of clozapine (which is a muscarinic antagonist), is itself actually an M1 agonist, and possibly a dopamine partial agonist. This compound is currently in testing in schizophrenia.

Cannabinoid antagonists. Cannabinoid receptors are linked to reward mechanisms in the mesolimbic system. An antagonist to cannabinoid 1 (CB1) receptors known as rimonabant, or SR141716 A, has been tested in schizophrenia, but without clearly improving psychosis. However, rimonabant is approved in some countries for obesity, as it may lead to weight loss; it is in testing also for smoking cessation and alcohol abuse. A related compound is SR 147778 (AVE 1625). Testing of rimonabant as a weight-loss agent in obesity has not yet been extensively completed for schizophrenic patients taking antipsychotics, but it could be an important intervention in reducing obesity and cardiometabolic risk in these patients.

Peptide-linked mechanisms

Neurokinin antagonists (NK1, NK2, and NK3). Testing with NK1 antagonists (also known as substance P antagonists) has generally been disappointing for all psychiatric indications, from schizophrenia to depression to pain. Testing with an NK2 antagonist for depression is promising. Finally, testing of various NK3 antagonists is in progress but without as yet any clear results of efficacy in schizophrenia. These drugs include talnetant (SB223412), osanetant (SR142801), SSR 146977, and the NK3/NK2 antagonist SR 241586.

Neurotensin antagonists. Neurotensin is a peptide neurotransmitter that is colocalized with dopamine in the mesolimbic dopamine pathway, but is much lower in concentration in nigrostriatal and mesocortical dopaminergic pathways. A nonpeptide antagonist SR-142948 is in clinical testing in schizophrenia as a theoretical agent that could reduce positive symptoms without producing EPS by exploiting differential actions on the mesolimbic rather than nigrostriatal dopamine systems; it has thus far not yielded definitive results.

Cholecystokinin. Cholecystokinin (CCK) is also colocalized with dopaminergic neurons and has two receptor subtypes, with CCK-A being predominantly outside the CNS and CCK-B within the CNS. Studies of CCK agonists and antagonists to date have not given clear clues as to their potential for therapeutic actions in schizophrenia.

Peptide treatments for obesity

Pramlintide. Pramlintide (Symlin) is a synthetic analog of the human peptide hormone amylin, a naturally occurring neuroendocrine hormone synthesized by pancreatic beta cells that contributes to glucose control during the postprandial period. Pramlintide is given at mealtimes as an adjunctive treatment to diabetics who fail to achieve desired glucose control despite adequate insulin (and oral hypoglycemic) therapy. It works by modulating gastric emptying, preventing the postprandial rise in plasma glucagon, and causing satiety, probably by a central mechanism leading to decreased caloric intake and potential weight loss. Thus it is being tested for obesity in general and – given the high incidence of obesity, cardiometabolic risk, and complications in schizophrenia – should be tested in schizophrenic patients taking atypical antipsychotic drugs.

Future combination chemotherapies for schizophrenia and other psychotic disorders

Given the economic incentives for providing the "cure" and treatment of choice for psychotic disorders, it is not difficult to understand why most drug development activities for the psychoses target a single disease mechanism with the goal of being the only therapy for a given disorder. In reality, it is overly simplistic to conceptualize disorders with psychotic features as the product of a single disease mechanism. Schizophrenia has not only psychotic features but also negative symptoms, affective symptoms, cognitive symptoms, and probably neurodevelopmental and neurodegenerative dimensions. It is difficult to conceptualize how such a complex disorder could ever be satisfactorily treated with a single entity acting by a single pharmacological mechanism.

Psychopharmacological treatments for schizophrenia in the future will need to borrow a chapter out of the book of cancer chemotherapy and HIV/AIDS therapy, where the standard of treatment is to use multiple drugs simultaneously to attain therapeutic synergy. "Combination chemotherapy" for malignancy utilizes the approach of combining several independent therapeutic mechanisms. When successful, this results in a total therapeutic response that is greater than the sum of its parts. This approach often has the favorable consequence of simultaneously diminishing total side effects, since adverse experiences of multiple drugs are mediated by different pharmacological mechanisms and therefore should not be additive. Clinical trials with multiple therapeutic agents working by several mechanisms can be quite difficult to undertake; but as there is a clinical trials methodology that exists in the cancer chemotherapy and HIV/AIDS literature, it is an approach that should be applied for complex disorders with multiple underlying disease mechanisms, such as schizophrenia. Thus, schizophrenia treatments of the near future will almost certainly combine new agents with one of the known atypical antipsychotics. Thus a platform of at least partial control of positive and negative symptoms, mood, cognition, and hostility will be provided with the known atypical antipsychotic, hopefully without causing EPS, tardive dyskinesia, hyperprolactinemia, or metabolic disturbances. New agents with new mechanisms can then "top up" the atypical antipsychotic, particularly in the hope of boosting the relief of negative and cognitive symptoms. In the long run, some sort of molecularly based therapy to prevent genetically programmed disease onset or progression or to reverse the consequences of aberrant neurodevelopment may also form part of the portfolio of treatments for schizophrenia.

Summary

This chapter has reviewed the pharmacology of conventional D2 antagonist antipsychotic drugs as well as the new atypical antipsychotic agents that are largely replacing them in clinical practice. The features of serotonin-2A/D2 antagonism (or SDA) of the atypical antipsychotic are discussed, as are several other pharmacological mechanisms that may contribute to atypical antipsychotic clinical actions, including D2 partial agonism (or DPA), rapid dissociation from D2 receptors, and serotonin-1A partial agonism (or SPA). Multiple receptor binding properties hypothesized to be linked to cardiometabolic risk and sedation of antipsychotics are explored. Pharmacokinetics of antipsychotics are briefly reviewed, as are the unique pharmacological and clinical properties of 15 specific antipsychotic agents. Use of these agents in a clinical practice setting, including considerations of how to treat individual symptoms of schizophrenia and how to dose, switch, and combine these agents for difficult patients are all reviewed. Finally, many new treatments under development for schizophrenia are presented.

Suggested Readings

Chapters 1 (Psychosis and Schizophrenia) and 2 (Antipsychotic Agents)

Abbatecola AM, Rizzo MR, Barbieri M, Grella R, Arciello A, Laieta MT, Acampora R, Passariello N, Cacciapuoti F and Paolisso G. (2006) Postprandial plasma glucose excursions and cognitive functioning in aged type 2 diabetics. *Neurology* 67; 7, 235–240.

Agid O, Mamo D, Ginovart N, Vitcu I, Wilson AA, Zipursky RB and Kapur S. (2007) Striatal vs extrastriatal dopamine D_2 receptors in antipsychotic response – a double-blind pet study in schizophrenia. *Neuropsychopharmacology* 32; 1209–1215.

Alphs LD, Summerfelt A, Lann H and Muller RJ. (1989) The negative symptom assessment: a new instrument to assess negative symptoms of schizophrenia. *Psychopharmacol Bull* 25; 2, 159–163.

Artaloytia JF, Arango C, Lahti A, Sanz J, Pascual A, Cubero P, Prieto D and Palomo T. (2006) Negative signs and symptoms secondary to antipsychotics: a double-blind, randomized trial of a single dose of placebo, haloperidol, and risperidone in healthy volunteers. *Am J Psychiatry* 163; 3, 488–493.

Atmaca M, Kuloglu M, Tezcan E and Ustundag B. (2003) Serum leptin and triglyceride levels in patients on treatment with atypical antipsychotics. *J Clin Psychiatry* 64; 5, 598–604.

Bai YM, Lin CC, Chen JY, Lin CY, Su TP and Chou P. (2006) Association of initial antipsychotic response to clozapine and long-term weight gain. *Am J Psychiatry* 163; 1276–1279.

Bardin L, Kleven MS, Barret-Grevoz C, Depoortere R and Newman-Tancredi A. (2006) Antipsychotic-like vs cataleptogenic actions in mice of novel antipsychotics having D2 antagonist and 5-HT1A agonist properties. *Neuropsychopharmacology* 31; 1869–1879.

Bennett S and Gronier B. (2005) Modulation of striatal dopamine release in vitro by agonists of the glycine_B site of NMDA receptors; interaction with antipsychotics. *Eur J Pharmacol* 527; 52–59.

Bota RG, Sagduyu K and Munro JS. (2005) Factors associated with the prodromal progression of schizophrenia that influence the course of the illness. *CNS Spectr* 10; 12, 937–942.

Bueller JA, Aftab M, Sen S, Gomez-Hassan D, Burmeister M and Zubieta JK. (2006) BDNF *Val*[66] *Met* allele is associated with reduced hippocampal volume in healthy subjects. *Biol Psychiatry* 59; 812–815.

Cannon TD, Glahn DC, Kim J, vanErp TGH, Karlsgodt K, Cohen MS, Neuchterlein KH, Bava S and Shirinyan D. (2005) Dorsolateral prefrontal cortex activity during maintenance and manipulation of information in working memory in patients with schizophrenia. *Arch Gen Psychiatry* 62; 1071–1080.

Cannon TD, Hennah W, van Erp TGM, Thompson PM, Lonnqvist J, Huttunen M, Gasperoni T, Tuulio-Henriksson T, Pirkola T, Toga AW, Kaprio J, Mazziotta J and Peltonen L. (2005) Association of DISC1(TRAX haplotypes with schizophrenia, reduced prefrontal gray matter, and impaired short- and long-term memory. *Arch Gen Psychiatry* 62; 1205–1213.

Chiu CC, Chen KP, Liu HC and Lu ML. (2006) The early effect of olanzapine and risperidone on insulin secretion in atypical-naïve schizophrenic patients. *J Clin Psychopharmacol* 26; 5, 504–507.

Citrome L, Jaffe A, Levine J and Martello D. (2006) Incidence, prevalence and surveillance for diabetes in New York State psychiatric hospitals, 1997–2004. *Psychiatr Serv* 57; 8, 1132–1139.

Citrome L, Macher JP, Salazar DE, Mallikaarjun S and Boulton DW. (2007) Pharmacokinetics of Aripiprazole and Concomitant Carbamazepine. *J Clin Psychopharmacol* 27; 3, 279–283.

Clinton SM, Ibrahim HM, Frey KA, Davis KL, Haroutunian V and Meador-Woodruff JH. (2005) Dopaminergic abnormalities in select thalamic nuclei in schizophrenia: involvement of the intracellular signal integrating proteins calcyon and spinophilin. *Am J Psychiatry* 162; 1859–1871.

Cornblatt BA, Lencz T, Smith CW, Olsen R, Auther AM, Nakayama E, Lesser ML, Tai JY, Shah MR, Foley CA, Kane JM and Correll CU. (2007) Can antidepressants be used to treat the schizophrenia prodrome? Results of a prospective, naturalistic treatment study of adolescents. *J Clin Psychiatry* 68; 4, 546–557.

Coyle JT and Tsai G. (2004) The NMDA receptor glycine modulatory site: a therapeutic target for improving cognition and reducing negative symptoms in schizophrenia. *Psychopharmacology* 174; 32–38.

Coyle JT, Tsai G and Goff D. (2003) Converging evidence of nmda receptor hypofunction in the pathophysiology of schizophrenia. *Ann N Y Acad Sci* 1003; 318–327.

Coyle JT. (2006) Glutamate and schizophrenia: beyond the dopamine hypothesis. *Cell Mol Neurobiol* 26; 4–6, 365–384.

Cropley VL, Fujita J, Innis RB and Nathan PJ. (2006) Molecular imaging of the dopaminergic system and its association with human cognitive function. *Biol Psychiatry* 59; 898–907.

De Bartolomeis A, Fiore G and Iasevoli F. (2005) Dopamine-glutamate interaction and antipsychotics mechanism of action: implication for new pharmacological strategies in psychosis. *Curr Pharm Design* 11; 351–3594.

Detera-Wadleigh SD and McMahon FJ. (2006) G72/G30 in schizophrenia and bipolar disorder: review and meta-analysis. *Biol Psychiatry* 60; 106–114.

DiForti M, Lappin JM and Murray RM. (2007) Risk factors for schizophrenia – all roads lead to dopamine. *Eur Neuropsychopharmacol* 17; S101–S107.

Emsley R, Rabinowitz J and Medori R. (2006) Time course for antipsychotic treatment response in first-episode schizophrenia. *Am J Psychiatry* 163; 743–745.

Essock SM, Covell NH, Davis SM, Stroup TS, Rosenheck RA and Lieberman JA. (2006) Effectiveness of switching antipsychotic medications. *Am J Psychiatry* 163; 12, 2090–2095.

Fanous AH, van den Oord EJ, Riley BP, Aggen SH, Neawle MC, O'Neill FA, Walsh D and Kendler KS. (2005) Relationship between a high-risk haplotype in the DTNBP1 (dysbindin) gene and clinical features of schizophrenia. *Am J Psychiatry* 162; 10, 1824–1832.

Fenton WS and Chavez MR. (2006) Medication-induced weight gain and dyslipidemia in patients with schizophrenia. *Am J Psychiatry* 163; 1697–1704.

Gilbert F, Morissette M, St-Hilaire M, Paquet B, Rouillard C, DiPaolo T and Levesque D. (2006) *Nur77* gene knockout alters dopamine neuron biochemical activity and dopamine turnover. *Biol Psychiatry* 60; 538–547.

Glenthoj BY, Mackeprang T, Svarer C, Rasmussen H, Pinborg LH, Friberg L, Baare W, Hemmingsen R and Videbaek C. (2006) Frontal dopamine $D_{2/3}$ receptor binding in drug-naïve first-episode schizophrenia patients correlates with positive psychotic symptoms and gender. *Biol Psychiatry* 60; 621–629.

Goldberg TE, Straub RE, Callicott JH, Hariri A, Mattay VS, Bigelow L, Coppola R, Egan MF and Weinberger DR. (2006) The G72/G30 gene complex and cognitive abnormalities in schizophrenia. *Neuropsychopharmacology* 31; 2022–2032.

Green EK, Raybould R, Macgregor S, Gordon-Smith K, Heron J, Hyde S, Grozeva D, Hamshere M, Williams N, Owen MJ, O'Donovan MC, Jones L, Jones I, Kirov G and Craddock N. (2005) Operation of the schizophrenia susceptibility gene, neuregulin 1, across traditional diagnostic boundaries to increase risk for bipolar disorder. *Arch Gen Psychiatry* 62; 642–648.

Green MF, Marder SR, Glynn SM, McGurk SR, Wirshing WC, Wirshing DA, Liberman RP and Mintz J. (2002) The neurocognitive effects of low-dose haloperidol: a two-year comparison with risperidone. *Biol Psychiatry* 51; 972–978.

Harrison PJ. (2007) Schizophrenia Susceptibility Genes and Neurodevelopment. *Biol Psychiatry* 61; 1119–1120.

Harrison PJ and Law AJ. (2006) Neuregulin 1 and schizophrenia: genetics, gene expression, and neurobiology. *Biol Psychiatry* 60; 132–140.

Henderson DC, Cagliero E, Copeland PM, Louie PM, Borba CP, Fan X, Freudenreich O and Goff DC. (2007) Elevated hemoglobin A1c as a possible indicator of diabetes mellitus and diabetic ketoacidosis in schizophrenia patients receiving atypical antipsychotics. *J Clin Psychiatry* 68; 533–541.

Heresco-Levy U, Bar G, Levin R, Ermilov M, Ebstein RP and Javitt DC. (2007) High glycine levels are associated with prepulse inhibition deficits in chronic schizophrenia patients. *Schizophr Res*, in press.

Heresco-Levy U, Javitt DC, Ebstein R, Vass Ag, Lichtenbwerg P, Bar G, Catinari S and Ermilov M. (2005) D-serine efficacy as add-on pharmacotherapy to risperidone and olanzapine for treatment-refractory schizophrenia. *Biol Psychiatry* 57; 577–585.

Ho BC, Milev P, O'Leary DS, Librant A and reasen NC and Wassink TH. (2006) Cognitive and magnetic resonance imaging brain morphometric correlates of brain-derived neurotrophic factor Val66Met gene polymorphism in patients with schizophrenia and healthy volunteers. *Arch Gen Psychiatry* 63; 731–740.

Houseknecht KL, Robertson AS, Zavadoski W, Gibbs EM, Johnson DE and Rollema H. (2007) Acute effects of atypical antipsychotics on whole-body insulin resistance in rats: implications for adverse metabolic effects. *Neuropsychopharmacology* 32; 289–297.

Hoyer D, Hannon JP and Martin GR. (2002) Molecular, pharmacological and functional diversity of 5-HT receptors. *Pharmacol Biochem Behav* 71; 533–554.

Hunter MD, Ganesan V, Wilkinson ID and Spence SA. (2006) Impact of modafinil on prefrontal executive function in schizophrenia. *Am J Psychiatry* 163; 12, 2184–2186.

Ingelman-Sundberg M. (2004) Pharmacogenetics of cytochrome P450 and its applications in drug therapy: the past, present and future. *Trends in Pharmacol Sci* 25; 4, 193–200.

Ishizuka K, Paek M, Kamiya A and Sawa A. (2006) A review of disrupted-in-schizophrenia-1 (disc1): neurodevelopment, cognition, and mental conditions. *Biol Psychiatry* 59; 1189–1197.

Javitt DC. (2006) Is the glycine site half saturated or half unsaturated? Effects of glutamatergic drugs in schizophrenia patients. *Curr Opin Psychiatry* 19; 151–157.

Javitt DC, Balla A, Burch S, Suckow R, Xie S and Sershen H. (2004) Reversal of phencyclidine-induced dopaminergic dysregulation by N-methyl-d-aspartate receptor/glycine-site agonists. *Neuropsychopharmacology* 29; 300–307.

Javitt DC, Duncan L, Balla A and Sershen H. (2005) Inhibition of system A-mediated glycine transport in cortical synaptosomes by therapeutic concentrations of clozapine: implications for mechanisms of action. *Mol Psychiatry* 10; 276–286.

Jindal RD and Keshavan S. (2006) Critical role of M_3 muscarinic receptor in insulin secretion. *J Clin Psychopharmacol* 26; 5, 449–450.

Johnson DE, Yamazaki H, Ward KM, Schmidt AW, Lebel WS, Treadway JL, Gibbs, EM, Zawalich WS and Rollema H. (2005) Inhibitory effects of antipsychotics on carbachol-enhanced insulin secretion from perifused rat islets. *Diabetes* 54; 1552–1558.

Johnson MR, Morris NA, Astur RS, Calhoun VD, Mathalon DH, Kiehl KA and Pearlson GD. (2006) A functional magnetic resonance imaging study of working memory abnormalities in schizophrenia. *Biol Psychiatry* 60; 11–21.

Jones PB, Barnes TRE, Davies L, Dunn G, Lloyd H, Hayhurst KP, Murray RM, Markwick A and Lewis SW. (2006) Randomized controlled trial of the effect on quality of life of second- vs first-generation antipsychotic drugs in schizophrenia. *Arch Gen Psychiatry* 63; 1079–1087.

Kahn RS, Schulz SC, Palazov VD, Reyes EB, Brecher M, Svensson O, Andersson HM and Meulien D. (2007) Efficacy and tolerability of once daily extended release quetiapine fumarate in acute schizophrenia: a randomized, double blind, placebo controlled study. *J Clin Psychiatry* 68; 6, 832–842.

Kalkman HO, Feuerbach D, Lotscher E and Schoeffter P. (2003) Functional characterization of the novel antipsychotic iloperidone at human D_2, D_3, Alpha$_{2c}$, 5-HT$_6$ and 5-HT$_{1A}$ receptors. *Life Sci* 73; 1151–1159.

Kapur S and Lecrubier Y. (eds) (2003) *Dopamine in the Pathophysiology and Treatment of Schizophrenia*. London, Martin Dunitz.

Kapur S. (2003) Psychosis as a state of aberrant salience: a framework linking biology, phenomenology, and pharmacology in schizophrenia. *Am J Psychiatry* 160; 1, 13–23.

Keefe RSE, Bilder RM, Davis SM, Harvey PD, Palmer BW, Gold JM, Meltzer HY, Green MF, Capuao G, Stroup TS, McEvoy JP, Swartz MS, Rosenheck RA, Perkins DO, Davis CE, Hsiao JK and Lieberman JA. (2007) Neurocognitive effects of antipsychotic medications in patients with chronic schizophrenia in the CATIE trial. *Arch Gen Psychiatry* 64; 633–647.

Keefe RSE, Bilder RM, Harvey PD, Davis SM, Palmer BW, Gold JM, Meltzer HY, Green MF, Miller DD, Canive JM, Adler LW, Manschreck TC, Swartz M, Rosenheck R, Perkins DO, Walker TM, Stroup TS, McEvoy JP and Lieberman JA. (2006) Baseline neurocognitive deficits in the CATIE schizophrenia trial. *Neuropsychopharmacology* 31; 2033–2046.

Keefe RSE, Seidman LJ, Christensen BK, Harner RM, Sharma T, Sitskoorn MM, Rock SL, Woolson S, Tohen M, Tollefson GD, Sanger TM and Lieberman JA. (2006) Long-Term neurocognitive effects of olanzapine or low-dose haloperidol in first episode psychosis. *Biol Psychiatry* 59; 97–105.

Kern RS, Green MF, Cornblatt BA, Owen JR, McQuade RD, Carson WH, Mirza A and Marcus R. (2006) The neurocognitive effects of aripiprazole: an open label comparison with olanzapine. *Psychopharmacology* 187; 312–320.

Kessler RM, Ansari MS, Riccardi P, Li R, Jayathilake K, Dawant B and Meltzer HY. (2006) Occupancy of striatal and extrastriatal dopamine D2 receptors by clozapine and quetiapine. *Neuropsychopharmacology* 31; 1991–2001.

Kessler RM, Ansari MS, Riccardi P, Li R, Jyathilake K, Dawant B and Meltzer JY. (2005) Occupancy of striatal and extrastriatal dopamine D2/D3 receptors by olanzapine and haloperidol. *Neuropsychopharmacology* 30; 2283–2289.

Klein DJ, Cottingham EM, Sorter M, Barton BA and Morrison JA. (2006) A randomized, double blind, placebo controlled trial of metformin treatment of weight gain associated with initiation of atypical antipsychotic therapy in children and adolescents. *Am J Psychiatry* 153; 2072–2079.

Lambert BL, Cunningham FE, Miller DR, Dalack GW and Hur K. (2006) Diabetes risk associated with use of olanzapine, quetiapine, and risperidon in Veterans health administration patients with schizophrenia. *Am J Epidemiol* 164; 672–681.

Lamberti JS, Olson D, Crilly JF, Olivares T, Williams GC, Tu X, Tang W, Wiener K, Dvorin S and Dietz MB. (2006) Prevalence of the metabolic syndrome among patients receiving clozapine. *Am J Psychiatry* 163; 1273–1276.

Lane HY, Chang YC, Liu YC, Chiu CC and Tsai GE. (2005) Sarcosine or D-Serine add-on treatment for acute exacerbation of schizophrenia. *Arch Gen Psychiatry* 62; 1196–1204.

Lane HY, Huang CL, Wu PL, Liu YC, Chang YC, Lin PY, Chen PW and Tsai G. (2006) Glycine Transporter 1 inhibitor, N-methylglycine (Sarcosine), added to clozapine for the treatment of schizophrenia. *Biol Psychiatry* 60; 645–649.

Lawler CP, Prioleau C, Lewis MM, Mak C, Jiang D, Schetz JA, Gonzalez AM, Sibley DR and Mailman RB. (1999) Interactions of the novel antipsychotic aripiprazole (OPC-14597) with dopamine and serotonin receptor subtypes. *Neuropsychopharmacology* 20; 6, 612–627.

Lencz T, Smith CW, McLaughlin D, Auther A, Nakayama E, Hovey L and Cornblatt BA. (2006) Generalized and specific neurocognitive deficits in prodromal schizophrenia. *Biol Psychiatry* 59; 863–871.

Leonard S and Freedman R. (2006) Genetics of chromosome 15q13-q14 in schizophrenia. *Biol Psychiatry* 60; 115–122.

Leucht S, Busch R, Math D, Kissling W and Kane JM. (2007) Early prediction of antipsychotic nonresponse among patients with schizophrenia. *J Clin Psychiatry* 68; 3, 352–360.

Levitt P, Ebert P, Mirnics K, Nimgaonkar VL and Lewis DA. (2006) Making the case for a candidate vulnerability gene in schizophrenia: convergent evidence for regulator of G-protein signaling 4 (RGS4). *Biol Psychiatry* 60; 534–537.

Lieberman JA, Tollefson GD, Charles, Zipursky R, Sharma T, Kahn RS, Keefe RSE, Green AI, Gur RE, McEvoy J, Perkins D, Hamer RM, Gu H and Tohen M. (2005) Antipsychotic drug effects on brain morphology in first episode psychosis. *Arch Gen Psychiatry* 62; 361–370.

Lindenmayer JP, Khan A, Iskander A, Abad MT and Parker B. (2007) A randomized controlled trial of olanzapine versus haloperidol in the treatment of primary negative symptoms and neurocognitive deficits in schizophrenia. *J Clin Psychiatry* 68; 3, 368–379.

Lipkovich I, Citrome L, Perlis R, Deberdt W, Jouston JP, Ahl J and Hardy T. (2006) Early predictors of substantial weight gain in bipolar patients treated with olanzapine. *J Clin Psychopharmocol* 26; 3, 316–320.

Liu YL, Fann SH, Liu CM, Chen WJ, Wu JY, Hung SI, Chen CH, Jou YSS, Liu SK, Hwang TJ, Hsieh MH, Ouyang WC, Chan HY, Chen JJ, Yang WC, Lin CY, Lee SFC and Hwu HG. (2006) A single nucleotide polymorphism fine mapping study of chromosome 1q42.1 reveals the vulnerability genes for schizophrenia, GNPAT and DISC1: association with impairment of sustained attention. *Biol Psychiatry* 60; 554–562.

Lovestone S, Killick R, DiFort M and Murry R. (2007) Schizophrenia as a GSK-3 dysregulation disorder. *Trends Neurosci* 30; 4, 142–149.

Lynch G and Gall CM. (2006) Ampakines and the threefold path to cognitive enhancement. *Trends Neurosci* 29; 10.

Maeda K, Nwulia E, Chang J, Balkissoon R, Ishizuka K, Chen H, Zandi P, McInnis MG and Sawa A. (2006) Differential expression of disrupted-in-schizophrenia (DISC1) in bipolar disorder. *Biol Psychiatry* 60; 929–935.

McCreary AD, Glennon JC, Ashby Jr R, Meltzer HY, Li Z, Reinders JH, Hesselink MB, Long SK, Herremans AH, van Stuivenberg H, Feenstra RW and Kruse CG. (2007) SLV313 (1-(2,3-dihydro-benzo[1,4] dioxin-5-yl)-4-[5-(4-fluoro-phenyl)-Pyridin-3-ylmethyl]-piperazine monohydrochloride): a novel dopamine D2 receptor Antagonist and 5-HT1A receptor agonist potential antipsychotic drug. *Neuropsychopharmacology* 32; 78–94.

McEvoy JP, Lieberman JA, Sroup TS, Davis SM, Meltzer HY, Rosenheck RA, Swartz MS, Perkins DO, Keefe, RSE, Davis CE, Severe J and Hsiao JK. (2006) Effectiveness of clozapine versus olanzapine, quetiapine, and risperidone in patients with chronic schizophrenia who did not respond to prior atypical antipsychotic treatment. *Am J Psychiatry* 163; 600–610.

McGlashan TH, Zipursky RB, Perkiins D, Addington J, Miller T, Woods SW, Hawkins KA, Hoffman RE, Predaw A and Epstein I. (2006) Randomized, double-blind trial of olanzapine versus placebo in patients prodromally symptomatic for psychosis. *Am J Psychiatry* 163; 790–799.

McLaughlin T, Abbasi F, Cheal K, Chu J, Lamendola C and Reaven G. (2003) Use of metabolic markers to identify overweight individuals who are insulin resistant. *Ann Intern Med* 139; 802–809.

Melle I, Johannesen JO, Friis S, Haahr U, Joa I, Larsen TK, Opjordsmoen S and Rund BR. (2006) Early detection of the first episode of schizophrenia and suicidal behavior. *Am J Psychiatry* 163; 5, 800–804.

Meyer-Lindenberg A, Buckholtz JW, Kolachana B, Hariri AR, Pezawas L, Blasi G, Wabnitz A, Honea R, Verchinski B, Callicott JH, Egan M, Mattay V and Weinberger DR. (2006) Neural mechanisms of genetic risk for impulsivity and violence in humans. *Proc Natl Acad Sci U S A* 103; 6, 6269–6274.

Meyer-Lindenberg A, Kohn PD, Kolachana B, Kippenhan S, McInerney-Leo A, Nussbaum R, Weinberger DR and Berman KF. (2005) Midbrain dopamine and prefrontal function in humans: interaction and modulation by COMT genotype. *Nat Neurosci* 8; 5, 594–596.

Millan MJ. (2005) N-Methyl-d-aspartate receptors as a target for improved antipsychotic agents: novel insights and clinical perspectives. *Psychopharmacology* 179; 30–53.

Mizrahi R, Rusjan P, Agid O, Graff A, Mamo DC, Zipursky RB and Kapur S. (2007) Adverse subjective experience with antipsychotics and its relationship to striatal and extrastriatal D2 receptors: a PET study in schizophrenia. *Am J Psychiatry* 164; 630–637.

Murphy BP, Chung YC, Park TW and McGorry PD. (2006) Pharmacological treatment of primary negative symptoms in schizophrenia: a systematic review. *Schizophr Res* 88; 5–25.

Natesan S, Reckless GE, Barlow KBL, Nobrega JN and Kapur S. (2007) Evaluation of N-desmethylclozapine as a potential antipsychotic – preclinical studies. *Neuropsychopharmacology* 32; 1540–1549.

Natesan S, Reckless GE, Nobrega JN, Fletcher PJ and Kapur S. (2006) Dissociation between in vivo occupancy and functional antagonism of dopamine D2 receptors: comparing aripiprazole to other antipsychotics in animal models. *Neuropsychopharmacology* 31; 1854–1863.

Newman-Trancredi A, Assie MB, Leduc N, Ormiere AM, Danty N and Cosi C. (2005) Novel antipsychotics activate recombinant human and native rat serotonin 5-HT1A receptors: affinity, efficacy and potential implications for treatment of schizophrenia. *Int J Neuropsychopharmacol* 8; 341–356.

Olfson M, Blanco C, Liu L, Moreno C and Laje G. (2006) National trends in the outpatient treatment of children and adolescents with antipsychotic drugs. *Arch Gen Psychiatry* 63; 679–685.

Olfson M, Marcus SC, Corey-Lisle P, Tuomari AV, Hines P and L'Italien GJ. (2006) Hyperlipidemia following treatment with antipsychotic medications. *Am J Psychiatry* 163; 1821–1825.

Olincy A, Harris JG, Johnson LL, Pender V, Kongs S, Allensworth D, Ellis J, Zerbe GO, Leonard S, Stevens KE, Stevens JO, Martin L, Adler LE, Soti F, Kem WR and Freedman R. (2006) Proof-of-concept trial of an alpha 7 nicotinic agonist in schizophrenia. *Arch Gen Psychiatry* 63; 630–638.

Osborn DPJ, Levy G, Nazareth I, Petersen I, Islam A and King MB. (2007) Relative risk of cardiovascular and cancer mortality in people with severe mental illness from the United Kingdom's general practice research database. *Arch Gen Psychiatry* 64; 242–249.

Passamonti L, Fera F, Magariello A, Cerasa A, Gioia MC, Muglia M, Nicoletti G, Gallo O, Provinciali L and Quattrone A. (2006) Monoamine oxidase-A genetic variations influence brain activity associated with inhibitory control: new insight into the neural correlates of impulsivity. *Biol Psychiatry* 59; 334–340.

Perkins DO, Gu H, Boteva K and Lieberman JA. (2005) Relationship between duration of untreated psychosis and outcome in first episode schizophrenia: a critical review and meta-analysis. *Am J Psychiatry* 162; 1785–1804.

Pierre JM, Peloian JH, Wirshing DA, Wirshing WC and Marder SR. (2007) A randomized, double-blind, placebo-controlled trial of modafinil for negative symptoms in schizophrenia. *J Clin Psychiatry* 68; 5, 705–710.

Polsky D, Doshi JA, Bauer MS and Glick HA. (2006) Clinical trial-based cost effectiveness analyses of antipsychotic use. *Am J Psychiatry* 163; 12, 2047–2056.

Porteous DJ, Thomson P, Brandon NJ and Millar JK. (2006) The genetics and biology of DISC1 – an emerging role in psychosis and cognition. *Biol Psychiatry* 60; 123–131.

Pralong E, Magistretti P and Stoop R. (2002) Cellular perspectives on the glutamate-monoamine interactions in limbic lobe structures and their relevance for some psychiatric disorders. *Prog Neurobiol* 67; 173–202.

Reaven G. (2004) The metabolic syndrome or the insulin resistance syndrome: different names, different concepts, and different goals. *Endocrinol Metab Clin North Am* 33; 283–303.

Reist C, Mintz J, Albers LJ, Jamas MM, Szabo S and Ozdemir V. (2007) Second-generation antipsychotic exposure and metabolic-related disorders in patients with schizophrenia. *J Clin Psychopharmacol* 27; 46–51.

Remington G, Mamo D, Labelle A, Reiss J, Shammi C, Mannaert E, Mann S and Kapur S. (2006) A PET study evaluating dopamine D_2 receptor occupancy for long-acting injectable risperidone. *Am J Psychiatry* 163; 3, 396–401.

Reyes M, Buitelaar J, Toren P, Augustyns I and Eerdekens M. (2006) A randomized, double-blind, placebo-controlled study of risperidone maintenance treatment in children and adolescents with disruptive behavior disorders. *Am J Psychiatry* 163; 402–410.

Reynolds GP, Yao Z, Zhang XB, Sun J and Zhang ZJ. (2004) Pharmacogenetics of treatment in first-episode schizophrenia: D3 and 5-HT2C receptor polymorphisms separately associate with positive and negative symptom response. *Eur Neuropsychopharmacol* 15; 143–151.

Rosenheck RA, Leslie DL, Sindelar J, Miller EA, Lin H, Stroup TS, McEvoy J, Davis SM, Keefe, RSE, Swartz M, Perkins DO, Hsiao JK and Lieberman J. (2006) Cost-effectiveness of second generation antipsychotics and perphenazine in a randomized trial of treatment for chronic schizophrenia. *Am J Psychiatry* 163; 12, 2080–2089.

Sacco KA, Termine A, Seyal A, Dudas MM, Vessicchio JC, Krishnan-Sarin S, Jatlow PI, Wexler BE and George TP. (2005) Effects of cigarette smoking on spatial working memory and attentional deficits in schziophrenia. *Arch Gen Psychiatry* 62; 649–659.

Sarafidis PA and Nilsson PM. (2006) The metabolic syndrome: a glance at its history. *J Hypertens* 24; 621–626.

Sarter M. (2006) Preclinical research into cognition enhancers. *Trends Pharmacol Sci* 27:11.

Scarr E, Beneyto M, Meador-Woodruff JH and Dean B. (2005) Cortical glutamatergic markers in schizophrenia. *Neuropsychopharmacology* 30; 1521–1531.

Sepehry AA, Potvin S, Elie R and Stip E. (2007) Selective serotonin reuptake inhibitor (SSRI) add-on therapy for the negative symptoms of schizophrenia: A meta-analysis. *J Clin Psychiatry* 68; 4, 604–610.

Shayegan DK and Stahl SM. (2005) Emotion processing, the amygdala, and outcome in schizophrenia. *Prog Neuropsychopharmacol Biol Psychiatry* 29; 840–845.

Simonson GD and Kendall DM. (2005) Diagnosis of insulin resistance and associated syndromes: the spectrum from the metabolic syndrome to type 2 diabetes mellitus. *Coron Artery Dis* 16; 465–472.

Smid P, Coolen HKAC, Keizer HG, van Hes R, de Moes JP, den Hartog AP, Stork B, Plekkenpol RH, Niemann LC, Stroomer CNJ, Tulp MTM, van Stuivenberg HH, McCreary AC, Hesselink M, Herremans AHJ and Kruse CG. (2005) Synthesis, structure-activity relationships, and biological properties of 1-heteroaryl-4-[ω-(1H-indol-3-yl) alkyl] piperazines, novel potential antipsychotics combining potent dopamine D2 receptor antagonism with potent serotonin reuptake inhibition. *J Med Chem* 48; 6855–6869.

Snitz BE, MacDonald III A, Cohen JD, Cho RY, Becker T and Carter CS. (2005) Lateral and medial hypofrontality in first-episode schizophrenia: functional activity in a medication-naïve state and effects of short-term atypical antipsychotic treatment. *Am J Psychiatry* 162; 12, 2322–2329.

Spurling RD, Lamberti JS, Olsen D, Tu X and Tang W. (2007) Changes in metabolic parameters with switching to aripiprazole from another second-generation antipsychotic: a retrospective chart review. *J Clin Psychiatry* 68; 3, 406–409.

Stahl SM. (2004) Prophylactic antipsychotics: do they keep you from catching schizophrenia? *J Clin Psychiatry* 65; 11, 1445–1446.

Stephan KE, Baldeweg T and Friston KJ. (2006) Synaptic plasticity and dysconnection in schizophrenia. *Biol Psychiatry* 59; 929–939.

Straub RE and Weinberger DR. (2006) Schizophrenia genes – famine to feast. *Biol Psychiatry* 60; 81–83.

Stroup TS, Lieberman JA, McEvoy JP, Swartz MS, Davis SM, Capuano GA, Rosenheck RA, Keefe RSE, Miller AL, Belz I and Hsiao JK. (2007) Effectiveness of olanzapine, quetiapine, and risperidone in patients with chronic schizophrenia after discontinuing perphenazine: a CATIE study. *Am J Psychiatry* 164; 415–427.

Surguladze S, Russell T, Kucharska-Pietura K, Travis MJ, Giampietro V, David AS and Philips ML. (2006) A reversal of the normal pattern of parahippocampal response to neutral and fearful faces is associated with reality distortion in schizophrenia. *Biol Psychiatry* 60; 423–431.

Takahashi H, Higuchi M and Suhara T. (2006) The role of extrastriatal dopamine D2 receptors in schizophrenia. *Biol Psychiatry* 59; 919–928.

Talkowski ME, Mansour H, Chowdari KV, Wood J, Butler A, Varma PG, Prasad S, Semwal P, Bhatia T, Deshpande S, Devlin B, Thelma BK and Nimgaonkar VL. (2006) Novel, replicated associations between dopamine D3 receptor gene polymorphisms and schizophrenia in two independent samples. *Biol Psychiatry* 60; 570–577.

Tarazi FI, Baldessarini RJ, Kula NS and Zhang K. (2003) Long-term effects of olanzapine, risperidone, and quetiapine on ionotropic glutamate receptor types: implications for antipsychotic drug treatment. *J Pharmacol Exp Ther* 306; 3, 1145–1151.

Tenback DE, van Harten PN, Sloof CJ and van Os J. (2006) Evidence that early extrapyramidal symptoms predict later tardive dyskinesia: a prospective analysis of 10,000 patients in the European schizophrenia outpatient health outcomes (SOHO) study. *Am J Psychiatry* 163; 1438–1440.

Tran-Johnson TK, Sack DA, Marcus RN, Auby P, McQuade RD and Oren DA. (2007) Efficacy and safety of intramuscular aripiprazole in patients with acute agitation: a randomized, double-blind, placebo-controlled trial. *J Clin Psychiatry* 68; 1, 111–119.

Tremeau F, Malaspina D, Duval F, Correa H, Hager-Budny M, Coin-Bariou L, Macher JP and Gorman JM. (2005) Facial expressiveness in patients with schizophrenia compared to depressed patients and nonpatient comparison subjects. *Am J Psychiatry* 162; 1, 92–101.

Tsai G, Lane HY, Chong MY and Lange N. (2004) Glycine transporter 1 inhibitor, N-methylglycine (sarcosine), added to antipsychotics for the treatment of schizophrenia. *Biol Psychiatry* 55; 452–456.

Tsai GE, Yang P, Chang YC and Chong MY. (2006) D-alanine added to antipsychotics for the treatment of schizophrenia. *Biol Psychiatry* 59; 230–234.

Tunbridge EM, Harrison PJ and Weinberger DR. (2006) Catechol-o-methyltransferase, cognition, and psychosis: Val[158] Met and beyond. *Biol Psychiatry* 60; 141–151.

Vestri HS, Maianu L, Moellering DR and Garvey WT. (2007) Atypical antipsychotic drugs directly impair insulin action in adipocytes: effects on glucose transport, lipogenesis, and antilipolysis. *Neuropsychopharmacology* 32; 765–772.

Vidalis AA. (2006) *Psychopharmacology Issues in Pregnancy and Lactation.* Thessasloniki, Greece, Contemporary Editions.

Voruganti Land Awad AG. (2004) Neuroleptic dysphoria: towards a new synthesis. *Psychopharmacology* 171; 121–132.

Walss-Bass C, Liu W, Lew DF, Villegas R, Montero P, Dassori A, Leach RJ, Almasy L, Escamilla M and Rawventos H. (2006) A novel missense mutation in the transmembrane domaine of neuregulin 1 is associated with schizophrenia. *Biol Psychiatry* 60; 548–553.

Weissman EM, Zhu CW, Schooler NR, Goetz RR and Essock SM. (2006) Lipid monitoring in patients with schizophrenia prescribed second generation antipsychotics. *J Clin Psychiatry* 67; 9, 1323–1326.

Wezenberg E, Verkes RJ, Ruigt GSF, Hulstijn W and Sabbe BGC. (2007) Acute effects of the ampakine farampator on memory and information processing in healthy elderly volunteers. *Neuropsychopharmacology* 32; 1272–1283.

Williams NM, Green EK, Macgregor S, Dwyer S, Norton N, Williams H, Raybould R, Grozeva D, Hamshere M, Zammit S, Jones L, Cardno A, Kirov G, Jones I, O'Donovan MC, Owen MJ and Craddock N. (2006) Variation at the DAOA/G30 locus influences susceptibility to major mood episodes but not psychosis in schizophrenia and bipolar disorder. *Arch Gen Psychiatry* 63; 366–373.

Winterer G, Egan MF, Kolachana BS, Goldberg TE, Coppola R and Weinberger DR. (2006) Prefrontal electrophysiologic noise and catechol-O-methyltransferase genotype in schizophrenia. *Biol Psychiatry* 60; 578–584.

Yaeger D, Smith HG and Altshuler LL. (2006) Atypical antipsychotics in the treatment of schizophrenia during pregnancy and the postpartum. *Am J Psychiatry* 163; 12, 2064–2070.

Zaboli G, Jonsson EG, Gizatullin R, Asberg M and Leopardi R. (2006) Tryptophan hydroxylase-1 gene variants associated with schizophrenia. *Biol Psychiatry* 60; 563–569.

Zhang M, Ballard ME, Kohlhaas KL, Browmna KE, Jongen-Relo AL, Unger LV, Fox GB, Gross G, Decker MW, Drescher KU and Rueter LE. (2006) Effect of dopamine D3 antagonists on PPI in DBA/2J mice or PPI deficit induced by neonatal ventral hippocampal lesions in rats. *Neuropsychopharmacology* 31; 1382–1392.

Index

Page numbers followed by '*f*' indicate figures; page numbers followed by '*t*' indicate tables.

amisulpride, 130, 134*f*, 135*f*, 176, 183
    and cardiometabolic risk, 140*t*
    clinical actions of, 125
    and diabetes, 171
    for negative symptoms in schizophrenia, 182*f*
    pharmacological icon, 177*f*
    and QTc prolongation, 171
amoxapine (Asendin), 173, 174*f*
AMPA (alpha-amino-3-hydroxy-5-methyl-4-
        isoxazole-priopionic acid) glutamate
        receptors, 64
    and synaptogenesis, 62
AMPA-kines, 199
amphetamines, 44
    and dopamine release, 26
    response to emotional input, 78
    and schizophrenia symptoms, 75, 77*f*
amylin, 204
anhedonia, 5, 6*t*, 30
antagonists,
    vs. inverse agonist, 105
    vs. partial agonists, 132*f*
    presynaptic, 199*f*
anticholinergic agents
    D2 antagonism and, 93*f*
    side effects, 95
antihistamines, 82
    atypical, 96
        administration frequency, 122
        cardiometabolic risk and, 140*t*
        cardiometabolic risk management, 145
        hit-and-run receptor binding properties,
            124*f*
        hypothetical action over time, 125*f*
        to improve schizophrenia symptoms, 109
        pharmacological properties, 139*f*
        and prolactin, 118*f*
        properties, 119, 135*f*
        and weight gain risk, 140*t*
    avoiding sedation and enhancing long-term
        outcome, 155*f*
    benzodiazepines to lead in or top off, 188*f*
    best practices for monitoring and managing,
        149*f*
    cardiometabolic risk and, 137–150
    combining two, 191
    conventional, 91*f*
        vs. atypical, 112*f*, 114*f*
        D2 binding of, 123*f*
        D2-receptor antagonist, 83
        hypothetical action over time, 123*f*
        muscarinic cholinergic blocking properties,
            91, 95
        pharmacological properties, 82–96

and prolactin, 118*f*
    risk and benefits of long-term, 95
    in use, 85*t*
as D2 dopamine receptor blockers, 27
first-generation, 83*f*, 96
high doses, 191*f*
links between binding properties and clinical
    actions, 136
low-potency, and dissociation, 124
"off-label" uses, 82
patient toleration of, 163
pharmacokinetics, 156–162
pharmacological properties, 162–179
prescribing information, 82
prophylactic, 192
receptor interactions for, 134
sedation as short-term tool, 152*f*
side effects and compliance, 153*f*
switching, 185, 187*f*
    process to avoid, 187*f*
    from sedating to nonsedating, 189*f*
antisocial personality disorder, 13
anxiety disorders
    5HT1A receptors and, 103*f*
    quetiapine for, 168*f*
anxious mood, 14
anxious self-punishment, 3
apathy, 3
    histamine-1 with 5HT2C antagonism, 141*f*
aripiprazole, 129, 130, 134*f*–136*f*, 158, 175, 183
    and cardiometabolic risk, 140*t*
    as CYP 2D6 substrate, 158, 159*f*
    and diabetes, 171
    dosage with carbamazepine, 161*f*, 162
    pharmacological icon, 176*f*
    raising levels of, 160*f*
    and sedation, 184, 186*f*
    switching from sedating agent to, 189
    and weight gain risk, 140*t*
aromatic amino acid decarboxylase (AAADC),
    97, 98*f*
asenapine, 122*f*, 200
Asendin (amoxapine), 173, 174*f*
asociality, 5, 6*t*
assaultiveness, 10
atorvastatin
    impaired, in schizophrenia, 11
attention deficit hyperactivity disorder
    (ADHD), 180
    symptoms shared with schizophrenia, 14
attitudes, hostile, 3
atypical antipsychotic agents, 96
    administration frequency, 122
    cardiometabolic risk and, 140*t*

extrapyramidal symptoms (EPS), 121, 123*f*
  5HT2A antagonist to reduce, 105, 107
  absence with atypical antipsychotics, 125*f*
  D2 receptor blockage and, 86
  dopamine partial agonism and, 132*f*
  risperidone and, 166
  from unwanted D2 receptor blockade, 136

fasting triglycerides
  antipsychotic agents and, 145*f*
  baseline measurement, 145, 149*f*
  monitoring, 150*f*
  quetiapine and, 169
  rapid elevation of, 141
  risperidone and, 167
  ziprasidone and, 171
fear. *See also* anxiety disorders
  processing by amygdala, 77*f*
    excitotoxicity in early development, 62*f*
    insult and schizophrenia, 57
    survival of wrong neurons, 59
  insults in neurodegenerative theories of
    schizophrenia, 54*f*
first-generation antipsychotic agents, 83*f*, 96
fluoxetine (Prozac),
  metabolite of, 159
  olanzapine and, 165
flupenthixol (Depixol), 85*t*
fluphenazine (Prolixin), 85*t*
fluvoxamine, 159, 200
free radicals, 60*f*
  and neuron death, 56
  scavengers for excitotoxicity, 196*f*

G protein-linked receptors, 103*f*
GABA (gamma-aminobutyric acid), 44*f*, 72*f*
GABA (gamma-aminobutyric acid) neurons,
  46, 47*f*
  for connecting serotonin and dopamine
    neurons, 105
  dopamine impact on, 48*f*
  release, 105*f*
galactorrhea, 32, 90
genes
  susceptibility, 58
    for schizophrenia, 63*t*, 73
genetic programming, in neurodegenerative
    theories of schizophrenia, 54*f*
glial alanine-serine-cysteine transporter
  (ASC-T), 34
  glutamine release from, 36*f*
  glycine from, 38
glial d-serine transporter, 38*f*
glial SNAT, 34, 36*f*, 38

glucose
  monitoring fasting, 146
  agonist actions at 5HT1A receptors and,
    131
  conversion to glutamine, 34, 35*f*
    system overactivity, 28, 55
  key pathways in brain, 43*f*, 41–45
    NMDA hypofunction hypothesis of
      schizophrenia and, 42–45
  NMDA receptor excitation spectrum by,
    57*f*
  pharmacology, 194
  preventing release, 199*f*
  recycled and regnerated, 35*f*
    conversion to glutamine, 36*f*
    glutamine release from glial cells, 36*f*
    5HT1A and 5HT2A receptor effect,
      115*f*
    regulation with 5HT1A, 113, 116
  role in schizophrenia pathophysiology, 33
  susceptibility gene effect on, 71
  synapses, convergence of susceptibility genes
    for schizophrenia on, 68
  synthesis, 33
glutamate receptors, 39, 40*f*
  metabotropic, 39, 42*f*
  types, 41*t*
glutamatergic corticostriatal projections,
    NMDA glutamate receptor
    hypofunction in, 51*f*
glutaminase, 34, 36*f*
glutamine
  glutamate conversion to, 34, 35*f*
  release from glial cells, 36*f*
glutamine synthetase, 34
glycine, 197, 197*f*
  from glial cells, 38
  from l-serine, 39
  production, 37
glycine agonists, 195
glycine transporters (GlyT1), 196
  inhibitors, 198*f*
grandiose expansiveness, 3
guilt, 14
  CYP450 enzymes in wall, 156
GW742457, 201

H1 histamine receptor, and weight gain, 137
hallucinations, 2, 5
  5HT2A receptors and, 103*f*
  5HT2A receptors effect on glutamate release
    and, 113
  antipsychotic action to reduce, 179
  mesolimbic dopamine pathway role in, 26